THE RESURGENCE OF BREASTFEEDING, 1975–2000

The transcript of a Witness Seminar held by the Wellcome Trust Centre for the History of Medicine at UCL, London, on 24 April 2007

Edited by S M Crowther, L A Reynolds and E M Tansey

Volume 35   2009

©The Trustee of the Wellcome Trust, London, 2009

First published by the Wellcome Trust Centre
for the History of Medicine at UCL, 2009

The Wellcome Trust Centre for the History of Medicine
at UCL is funded by the Wellcome Trust, which is
a registered charity, no. 210183.

ISBN 978 085484 119 6

All volumes are freely available online following the links to Publications/Wellcome Witnesses at
www.ucl.ac.uk/histmed

Technology Transfer in Britain: The case of monoclonal antibodies; Self and Non-Self: A history of autoimmunity; Endogenous Opiates; The Committee on Safety of Drugs • Making the Human Body Transparent: The impact of NMR and MRI; Research in General Practice; Drugs in Psychiatric Practice; The MRC Common Cold Unit • Early Heart Transplant Surgery in the UK • Haemophilia: Recent history of clinical management • Looking at the Unborn: Historical aspects of obstetric ultrasound • Post Penicillin Antibiotics: From acceptance to resistance? • Clinical Research in Britain, 1950–1980 • Intestinal Absorption • Origins of Neonatal Intensive Care in the UK • British Contributions to Medical Research and Education in Africa after the Second World War • Childhood Asthma and Beyond • Maternal Care • Population-based Research in South Wales: The MRC Pneumoconiosis Research Unit and the MRC Epidemiology Unit • Peptic Ulcer: Rise and fall • Leukaemia • The MRC Applied Psychology Unit • Genetic Testing • Foot and Mouth Disease: The 1967 outbreak and its aftermath • Environmental Toxicology: The legacy of Silent Spring • Cystic Fibrosis • Innovation in Pain Management • The Rhesus Factor and Disease Prevention • The Recent History of Platelets in Thrombosis and Other Disorders • Short-course Chemotherapy for Tuberculosis • Prenatal Corticosteroids for Reducing Morbidity and Mortality after Preterm Birth • Public Health in the 1980s and 1990s: Decline and rise? • Cholesterol, Atherosclerosis and Coronary Disease in the UK, 1950–2000 • Development of Physics Applied to Medicine in the UK, 1945–90 • The Early Development of Total Hip Replacement • The Discovery, Use and Impact of Platinum Salts as Chemotherapy Agents for Cancer • Medical Ethics Education in Britain, 1963–1993 • Superbugs and Superdrugs: A history of MRSA • Clinical Pharmacology in the UK, c. 1950–2000: Influences and institutions • Clinical Pharmacology in the UK, c. 1950–2000: Industry and regulation • The Resurgence of Breastfeeding, 1975–2000

CONTENTS

ILLUSTRATIONS AND CREDITS

ABBREVIATIONS

COMA	Committee on Medical Aspects of Food and Nutrition Policy (DHSS)
DoH	Department of Health
DHSS	Department of Health and Social Security
FAO	Food and Agricultural Organization
HRP	Human Reproduction Programme
IBFAN	International Baby Food Action Network
ISRHML	International Society of Research in Human Milk and Lactation
LAM	Lactation Amenorrhea Method (of contraception)
LLLI	La Leche League International
LLLGB	La Leche League Great Britain
NCT	National Childbirth Trust
NICE	National Institute for Health and Clinical Excellence
ONS	Office for National Statistics
OPCS	Office of Population Censuses and Surveys
PAG	Protein-Calorie Advisory Group of the United Nations System
RDA	Recommended Dietary Allowances
UNICEF	United Nations International Children's Emergency Fund
WABA	World Alliance for Breastfeeding Action
WHO	World Health Organization

WITNESS SEMINARS:
MEETINGS AND PUBLICATIONS[1]

In 1990 the Wellcome Trust created a History of Twentieth Century Medicine Group, associated with the Academic Unit of the Wellcome Institute for the History of Medicine, to bring together clinicians, scientists, historians and others interested in contemporary medical history. Among a number of other initiatives the format of Witness Seminars, used by the Institute of Contemporary British History to address issues of recent political history, was adopted, to promote interaction between these different groups, to emphasize the potential benefits of working jointly, and to encourage the creation and deposit of archival sources for present and future use. In June 1999 the Governors of the Wellcome Trust decided that it would be appropriate for the Academic Unit to enjoy a more formal academic affiliation and turned the Unit into the Wellcome Trust Centre for the History of Medicine at UCL from 1 October 2000. The Wellcome Trust continues to fund the Witness Seminar programme via its support for the Centre.

The Witness Seminar is a particularly specialized form of oral history, where several people associated with a particular set of circumstances or events are invited to come together to discuss, debate, and agree or disagree about their memories. To date, the History of Twentieth Century Medicine Group has held more than 50 such meetings, most of which have been published, as listed on pages xiii–xxi.

Subjects are usually proposed by, or through, members of the Programme Committee of the Group, which includes professional historians of medicine, practising scientists and clinicians, and once an appropriate topic has been agreed, suitable participants are identified and invited. This inevitably leads to further contacts, and more suggestions of people to invite. As the organization of the meeting progresses, a flexible outline plan for the meeting is devised, usually with assistance from the meeting's chairman, and some participants are invited to 'set the ball rolling' on particular themes, by speaking for a short period to initiate and stimulate further discussion.

---

[1] The following text also appears in the 'Introduction' to recent volumes of *Wellcome Witnesses to Twentieth Century Medicine* published by the Wellcome Trust and the Wellcome Trust Centre for the History of Medicine at UCL.

Each meeting is fully recorded, the tapes are transcribed and the unedited transcript is sent to every participant. Each is asked to check his or her own contributions and to provide brief biographical details. The editors turn the transcript into readable text, and participants' minor corrections and comments are incorporated into that text, while biographical and bibliographical details are added as footnotes, as are more substantial comments and additional material provided by participants. The final scripts are then sent to every contributor, accompanied by forms assigning copyright to the Wellcome Trust. Copies of all additional correspondence received during the editorial process are deposited with the records of each meeting in archives and manuscripts, Wellcome Library, London.

As with all our meetings, we hope that even if the precise details of some of the technical sections are not clear to the non-specialist, the sense and significance of the events will be understandable. Our aim is for the volumes that emerge from these meetings to inform those with a general interest in the history of modern medicine and medical science; to provide historians with new insights, fresh material for study, and further themes for research; and to emphasize to the participants that events of the recent past, of their own working lives, are of proper and necessary concern to historians.

ACKNOWLEDGEMENTS

'The resurgence of breastfeeding, *c.* 1975-2000' was suggested as a suitable topic for a witness seminar by Professor Lawrence Weaver, who assisted us in planning the meeting. We are very grateful to him for his input and for his excellent chairing of the occasion. We are particularly grateful to Professor Rima Apple for writing such a useful Introduction to these published proceedings. We thank Mr James Akre, Professor Lars Hanson, Mrs Rachel O'Leary, Dr Felicity Savage and Professor Lawrence Weaver for their help with the Glossary and Dr Elisabet Helsing, Mrs Patti Rundall, Dr Felicity Savage, Miss Chloe Fisher, Professor Roger Short, Dr Anthony Williams and Mr John Wells for help with illustrations. For permission to reproduce images included here, we thank the World Alliance for Breastfeeding Action, Healthlink Worldwide, the Wellcome Trust and Cow and Gate.

As with all our meetings, we depend a great deal on our colleagues at the Wellcome Trust to ensure their smooth running: the Audiovisual Department, and the Medical Photographic Library; Mr Akio Morishima, who has supervised the design and production of this volume; our indexer, Ms Liza Furnival; and our readers, Mrs Sarah Beanland and Mr Simon Reynolds; Mrs Jaqui Carter is our transcriber, and Mrs Wendy Kutner and Dr Daphne Christie assisted us in running this meeting. Finally we thank the Wellcome Trust for supporting this programme.

Tilli Tansey

Lois Reynolds

Stefania Crowther

Wellcome Trust Centre for the History of Medicine at UCL

HISTORY OF TWENTIETH CENTURY MEDICINE WITNESS SEMINARS, 1993–2008

PUBLISHED MEETINGS

'…Few books are so intellectually stimulating or uplifting'.
Journal of the Royal Society of Medicine (1999) **92:** 206–8,
review of vols 1 and 2

'…This is oral history at its best…all the volumes make compulsive reading…they are, primarily, important historical records'.
British Medical Journal (2002) **325:** 1119, review of the series

Technology transfer in Britain: The case of monoclonal antibodies
Self and non-self: A history of autoimmunity
Endogenous opiates
The Committee on Safety of Drugs
Tansey E M, Catterall P P, Christie D A, Willhoft S V, Reynolds L A. (eds)
(1997) *Wellcome Witnesses to Twentieth Century Medicine.* Volume 1. London:
The Wellcome Trust, 135pp. ISBN 1 869835 79 4

Making the human body transparent: The impact of NMR and MRI
Research in general practice
Drugs in psychiatric practice
The MRC Common Cold Unit
Tansey E M, Christie D A, Reynolds L A. (eds) (1998) *Wellcome
Witnesses to Twentieth Century Medicine.* Volume 2. London: The Wellcome
Trust, 282pp. ISBN 1 869835 39 5

Early heart transplant surgery in the UK
Tansey E M, Reynolds L A. (eds) (1999) *Wellcome Witnesses to
Twentieth Century Medicine.* Volume 3. London: The Wellcome Trust, 72pp.
ISBN 1 841290 07 6

Haemophilia: Recent history of clinical management
Tansey E M, Christie D A. (eds) (1999) *Wellcome Witnesses to
Twentieth Century Medicine.* Volume 4. London: The Wellcome Trust, 90pp.
ISBN 1 841290 08 4

Looking at the unborn: Historical aspects of obstetric ultrasound
Tansey E M, Christie D A. (eds) (2000) *Wellcome Witnesses to
Twentieth Century Medicine.* Volume 5. London: The Wellcome Trust, 80pp.
ISBN 1 841290 11 4

Post penicillin antibiotics: From acceptance to resistance?
Tansey E M, Reynolds L A. (eds) (2000) *Wellcome Witnesses to Twentieth Century Medicine.* Volume 6. London: The Wellcome Trust, 71pp. ISBN 1 841290 12 2

Clinical research in Britain, 1950–1980
Reynolds L A, Tansey E M. (eds) (2000) *Wellcome Witnesses to Twentieth Century Medicine.* Volume 7. London: The Wellcome Trust, 74pp. ISBN 1 841290 16 5

Intestinal absorption
Christie D A, Tansey E M. (eds) (2000) *Wellcome Witnesses to Twentieth Century Medicine.* Volume 8. London: The Wellcome Trust, 81pp. ISBN 1 841290 17 3

Neonatal intensive care
Christie D A, Tansey E M. (eds) (2001) *Wellcome Witnesses to Twentieth Century Medicine.* Volume 9. London: The Wellcome Trust Centre for the History of Medicine at UCL, 84pp. ISBN 0 854840 76 1

British contributions to medical research and education in Africa after the Second World War
Reynolds L A, Tansey E M. (eds) (2001) *Wellcome Witnesses to Twentieth Century Medicine.* Volume 10. London: The Wellcome Trust Centre for the History of Medicine at UCL, 93pp. ISBN 0 854840 77 X

Childhood asthma and beyond
Reynolds L A, Tansey E M. (eds) (2001) *Wellcome Witnesses to Twentieth Century Medicine.* Volume 11. London: The Wellcome Trust Centre for the History of Medicine at UCL, 74pp. ISBN 0 854840 78 8

Maternal care
Christie D A, Tansey E M. (eds) (2001) *Wellcome Witnesses to Twentieth Century Medicine.* Volume 12. London: The Wellcome Trust Centre for the History of Medicine at UCL, 88pp. ISBN 0 854840 79 6

Population-based research in south Wales: The MRC Pneumoconiosis Research Unit and the MRC Epidemiology Unit
Ness A R, Reynolds L A, Tansey E M. (eds) (2002) *Wellcome Witnesses to Twentieth Century Medicine.* Volume 13. London: The Wellcome Trust Centre for the History of Medicine at UCL, 74pp. ISBN 0 854840 81 8

The Rhesus factor and disease prevention
Zallen D T, Christie D A, Tansey E M. (eds) (2004) *Wellcome Witnesses to Twentieth Century Medicine.* Volume 22. London: The Wellcome Trust Centre for the History of Medicine at UCL, 98pp. ISBN 0 85484 099 0

The recent history of platelets in thrombosis and other disorders
Reynolds L A, Tansey E M. (eds) (2005) *Wellcome Witnesses to Twentieth Century Medicine.* Volume 23. London: The Wellcome Trust Centre for the History of Medicine at UCL, 186pp. ISBN 0 85484 103 2

Short-course chemotherapy for tuberculosis
Christie D A, Tansey E M. (eds) (2005) *Wellcome Witnesses to Twentieth Century Medicine.* Volume 24. London: The Wellcome Trust Centre for the History of Medicine at UCL, 120pp. ISBN 0 85484 104 0

Prenatal corticosteroids for reducing morbidity and mortality after preterm birth
Reynolds L A, Tansey E M. (eds) (2005) *Wellcome Witnesses to Twentieth Century Medicine.* Volume 25. London: The Wellcome Trust Centre for the History of Medicine at UCL, 154pp. ISBN 0 85484 102 4

Public health in the 1980s and 1990s: Decline and rise?
Berridge V, Christie D A, Tansey E M. (eds) (2006) *Wellcome Witnesses to Twentieth Century Medicine.* Volume 26. London: The Wellcome Trust Centre for the History of Medicine at UCL, 101pp. ISBN 0 85484 106 7

Cholesterol, atherosclerosis and coronary disease in the UK, 1950–2000
Reynolds L A, Tansey E M. (eds) (2006) *Wellcome Witnesses to Twentieth Century Medicine.* Volume 27. London: The Wellcome Trust Centre for the History of Medicine at UCL, 164pp. ISBN 0 85484 107 5

Development of physics applied to medicine in the UK, 1945–90
Christie D A, Tansey E M. (eds) (2006) *Wellcome Witnesses to Twentieth Century Medicine.* Volume 28. The Wellcome Trust Centre for the History of Medicine at UCL, 141pp. ISBN 0 85484 108 3

Early development of total hip replacement
Reynolds L A, Tansey E M. (eds) (2007) *Wellcome Witnesses to Twentieth Century Medicine.* Volume 29. London: The Wellcome Trust Centre for the History of Medicine at UCL, 198pp. ISBN 978 085484 111 0

The discovery, use and impact of platinum salts as chemotherapy agents for cancer
Christie D A, Tansey E M. (eds) (2007) *Wellcome Witnesses to Twentieth Century Medicine.* Volume 30. London: The Wellcome Trust Centre for the History of Medicine at UCL, 142pp. ISBN 978 085484 112 7

Medical Ethics Education in Britain, 1963–93
Reynolds L A, Tansey E M. (eds) (2007) *Wellcome Witnesses to Twentieth Century Medicine.* Volume 31. London: The Wellcome Trust Centre for the History of Medicine at UCL, 241pp. ISBN 978 085484 113 4

Superbugs and superdrugs: A history of MRSA
Reynolds L A, Tansey E M. (eds) (2008) *Wellcome Witnesses to Twentieth Century Medicine.* Volume 32. London: The Wellcome Trust Centre for the History of Medicine at UCL, 167pp. ISBN 978 085484 114 1

Clinical pharmacology in the UK, *c.* 1950–2000: Influences and institutions
Reynolds L A, Tansey E M. (eds) (2008) *Wellcome Witnesses to Twentieth Century Medicine.* Volume 33. London: The Wellcome Trust Centre for the History of Medicine at UCL, 148pp. ISBN 978 085484 117 2

Clinical pharmacology in the UK, *c.* 1950–2000: Industry and regulation
Reynolds L A, Tansey E M. (eds) (2008) *Wellcome Witnesses to Twentieth Century Medicine.* Volume 34. London: The Wellcome Trust Centre for the History of Medicine at UCL, 168pp. ISBN 978 085484 118 9

The resurgence of breastfeeding, 1975–2000
Crowther S M, Reynolds L A, Tansey E M. (eds) (2009) *Wellcome Witnesses to Twentieth Century Medicine.* Volume 35. London: The Wellcome Trust Centre for the History of Medicine at UCL (this volume). ISBN 978 085484 119 6

The development of sports medicine in twentieth century Britain
Reynolds L A, Tansey E M. (eds) (2009) *Wellcome Witnesses to Twentieth Century Medicine.* Volume 36. London: The Wellcome Trust Centre for the History of Medicine at UCL (in press). ISBN 978 085484 121 9

History of dialysis in the UK: *c.* 1950–2000
Crowther S M, Reynolds L A, Tansey E M. (eds) (2009) *Wellcome Witnesses to Twentieth Century Medicine.* Volume 37. London: The Wellcome Trust Centre for the History of Medicine at UCL (in press). ISBN 978 085484 122 6

History of cervical cancer and the role of the human papillomavirus over the last 25 years
Reynolds L A, Tansey E M. (eds) (2009) *Wellcome Witnesses to Twentieth Century Medicine.* Volume 38. London: The Wellcome Trust Centre for the History of Medicine at UCL (in press). ISBN 978 085484 123 3

Hard copies of volumes 1–20 are now available for free, while stocks last. We would be happy to send complete sets to libraries in developing or restructuring countries. Available from Dr Carole Reeves at: c.reeves@ucl.ac.uk

All volumes are freely available online at www.ucl.ac.uk/histmed/ publications/wellcome-witnesses/index.html or by following the links to Publications/Wellcome Witnesses at www.ucl.ac.uk/histmed

A hard copy of volumes 21–35 can be ordered from www.amazon.co.uk; www.amazon.com; and all good booksellers for £6/$10 plus postage, using the ISBN.

OTHER PUBLICATIONS

Technology transfer in Britain: The case of monoclonal antibodies
In: Tansey E M, Catterall P P. (1993) *Contemporary Record* **9**: 409–44.

Monoclonal antibodies: A witness seminar on contemporary medical history
In: Tansey E M, Catterall P P. (1994) *Medical History* **38**: 322–7.

Chronic pulmonary disease in South Wales coalmines: An eye-witness account of the MRC surveys (1937–42)
In: D'Arcy Hart P, edited and annotated by E M Tansey. (1998) *Social History of Medicine* **11**: 459–68.

Ashes to Ashes – The history of smoking and health
In: Lock S P, Reynolds L A, Tansey E M. (eds) (1998) Amsterdam: Rodopi BV, 228pp. ISBN 90420 0396 0 (Hfl 125) (hardback). Reprinted 2003.

Witnessing medical history. An interview with Dr Rosemary Biggs
Professor Christine Lee and Dr Charles Rizza (interviewers). (1998) *Haemophilia* **4**: 769–77.

Witnessing the Witnesses: Pitfalls and potentials of the Witness Seminar in twentieth century medicine
By E M Tansey. In: Doel R, Soderqvist T. (eds) (2006) *Writing Recent Science: The historiography of contemporary science, technology and medicine.* London: Routledge, 260–78.

The Witness Seminar technique in modern medical History of Medicine
By E M Tansey. In: Cook H J, Bhattacharya S, Hardy A. (eds) (2009) *History of the Social Determinants of Health: Global histories, contemporary debates.* London: Orient BlackSwan, 279–95.

INTRODUCTION

For millennia, infant feeding was breastfeeding and the nursing mother was idealized as the source of strength, of power, of family. Before the nineteenth century, infants denied breast-milk were not likely to survive. Medicine could provide a substitute for mother's milk, if absolutely necessary, but artificial feeding was a poor substitute for breastfeeding. Yet, by the middle of the twentieth century, in many industrialized countries, the overwhelming majority of infants were bottle-fed. In a popular 1957 childcare book, the chapter titled 'Breastfeeding' opens with the question: 'Breast or bottle?' and answers: 'This is something that every mother must decide for herself.'[2] The good doctor–author explains that a mother might choose not to breastfeed for many reasons: if she has tuberculosis; if she has had serious complications from labour; if her breast is infected; and if she 'dislikes the idea of nursing'. Moreover, he assures the reader that:

> A mother who cannot or does not wish to nurse, or a mother who must return to a job should not feel that she is neglecting an important duty… A bottle mother may still be a perfect mother.[3]

With developments in science, in clinical medicine and in commerce, with changes in women's roles in society and with the increasing concern over the high rates of infant mortality and morbidity, by the first half of the twentieth century, clinicians and researchers all agreed that 'breast is best'. At the same time, however, they insisted that with modern medicine, modern technology, clean water and a careful mother, bottle-feeding was satisfactory for most infants.

Mid-nineteenth-century medical science had generated increasingly sophisticated analyses of milk – human milk, goats' milk, cows' milk and mares' milk. Cows' milk and human milk differed in more than chemical composition. Nursing mothers and wet-nurses fed their infants directly from the breast, whereas cows' milk, especially that sold in cities, passed through many hands and the product bought by the consumer was often not pure. In addition, by the 1870s, those aware of contemporary bacteriological research also worried about bacterial contamination. To eliminate these problems doctors recommended heating the milk. As physicians determined the differences among milks, they worked to create a suitable match for human milk.

---

[2] Holt (1957): 63.

[3] Holt (1957): 65.

By late in the century, extremely high infant mortality rates alarmed the general public and galvanized medical researchers, who declared that the most significant cause of infant deaths was poor diet. As Thomas Morgan Rotch, a leading pediatrician and Harvard professor at the turn of the century stated:

> The preventive medicine of early life is pre-eminently the intelligent management of the nutriment which enables young human beings to breathe and grow and live. In fact, it is a proper or improper nutriment which makes or mars the perfection of the coming race. Infant feeding, then, is the subject of all others which should interest and incite to research all who are working in the preventive medicine of early life.[4]

Infant feeding studies became the raison d'être of paediatric research and increasingly infant feeding became the focus of paediatric practice, too.

In addition to physicians, manufacturers also sought to create a substitute for human milk. Some of these products, such as Liebig's Food, which was concocted by Justus Liebig in the 1860s, were intended to be dissolved in milk. Others, such as Nestlé's Milk Food, were complete foods, already containing milk. These products flooded the market in the second half of the nineteenth century, widely advertised in medical journals to physicians, and women's and general interest magazines to mothers.

Women were aware of the higher mortality rates for bottle-fed infants, yet not every mother could or would nurse her child. Allegedly, increasing numbers of women refused to breastfeed because nursing 'tied them down', as changes in modern society not only altered women's domestic roles but also extended their activities outside the home. Though few women voiced this sentiment themselves, no doubt some mothers felt constrained when they had to stay at home to nurse an infant. Other women worried that their milk supplies were inadequate, believing that physical conditions and the effects of modern life could prevent successful lactation. Such women wanted a convenient, safe and healthful alternative to mother's milk. They looked to science for the solution.

By the 1920s, bottle-feeding had become the generally accepted mode of infant feeding. Physicians and other commentators continued to give lip-service to the benefits of breast-milk, but they were willing and sometimes eager to replace the mother's breast with a bottle. As one mother related in 1926:

---

[4] Rotch (1893): 505.

I have a fine baby boy, age 12 weeks, weight 12 pounds 6 oz. At first I had more than enough milk for him but the last two weeks I have not had enough, and had my doctor give me a formula for to feed him part time – about two or three feedings a day. I do not understand why I cannot nurse him as at first…. When I asked my doctor again about it, he said: 'Why don't you wean him altogether?'[5]

With a bottle one could be certain of what the infant was receiving, both qualitatively and quantitatively. Moreover, products such as SMA and Nestlé's were fortified with newly discovered and synthesized vitamins, which promised protection against diseases such as rickets. When paediatric researchers conducted studies comparing the health of breast- and bottle-fed babies, they concluded that there was little difference in their health status, if the mother followed carefully the rules laid out by her physician for feeding the child.

Another significant factor that promoted artificial infant feeding in the twentieth century in developed countries was the increasingly common practice of hospitalized childbirth. These institutions provided a prime educational situation for isolated, nervous mothers who looked to modern, scientific childcare to ensure the health of their families. As hospitalized childbirth became increasingly popular, doctors and hospital administrators saw epidemics sweeping through their maternity wards. Our knowledge about the spread of diseases grew in the late nineteenth and early twentieth centuries when scientists and doctors developed a greater understanding of the germ theory of disease. However, knowledge of the transmission of disease did not immediately lead to knowledge about the prevention of disease. The era of sulfa drugs and antibiotics was decades away. Fearful of epidemics, hospitals would care for newborns in sterile nurseries, safely separated from their mothers who saw them only for feedings, every three or four hours. Visualize the typical situation of the twentieth-century new mother: for most of her 7–10 days in the hospital after childbirth she would peer through the window of the nursery looking at her child. Every several hours, a nurse would bring the baby to the mother, who carefully unwrapped the baby and tried to feed it. Within a few minutes, the nurse would be back to whisk the baby away again. These procedures left little time for the mother and baby to get acquainted or for the mother to feel comfortable caring for her child. Additionally, acting on the medical profession's concern about the initial weight loss exhibited by many newborns, hospitals

---

[5] Mrs C A, Detroit, Michigan, 2 March 1926, letter to the US Children's Bureau, quoted in Ladd-Taylor (1986): 77–8.

often instituted automatic supplemental feeding programmes. Nursing mothers were encouraged to sleep through the night and babies received night bottle-feedings in the nursery. Thus, hospital conditions and practices discouraged breastfeeding and encouraged the belief that bottle-feeding was as good as, if not better than, mother's milk.

Throughout the twentieth century, women in the developed world observed the benefits of modern medical science. When their children faced previously disastrous childhood diseases such as diphtheria and pneumonia, physicians treated them with new discoveries like diphtheria antitoxin, sulfa drugs and penicillin, and they thrived. Children who experienced nutritional deficiencies improved dramatically through the use of newly found and synthesized vitamins and other micronutrients. The manufacture of insulin enabled diabetic children to survive and to live healthy lives. Consequently, mothers concerned for the wellbeing of their families embraced bottle-feeding as the modern and scientific way to ensure the health of their infants.

Many of the same scientific, medical, commercial and social factors that had interested nineteenth-century physicians revived concerns about infant feeding in the late twentieth century. At the same time, observers recognized that there was a decline in maternal nursing in the developing world, a decline linked to a significant worsening of already high infant mortality rates. Many physicians, nurses, nutritionists and public health officials acknowledged this growing problem and turned once again to the study of mother's milk. Researchers scrutinized the parameters of maternal nursing with the goal of establishing the most healthful form of infant feeding. Given that breast-milk is best, for how long should an infant be breastfed? For how long should the infant be exclusively breastfed? What, if any, supplements are healthful? Necessary? Under what conditions, if any, should a mother forego breastfeeding her child? As in the earlier period, researchers also studied the mother's ability to produce appropriate breast-milk. Were some women unsuited for maternal nursing because of their nutritional status or other physical condition? The questions were similar to those posed a century earlier, but with newer, more sophisticated laboratory assays, more complex analyses integrating scientific, social, cultural and environmental factors, and more broadly drawn and clearly defined data bases, the interdisciplinary studies conducted by researchers and clinicians, as well as the participation of international agencies with their unavoidable political agendas, made breastfeeding a critical topic of discussion in medical and public health circles and brought renewed attention to those age-old questions.

As this Witness Seminar documents, the admonition that 'breast is best' is not a simple solution to the problem of infant mortality and morbidity. Maternal nursing is a complex physiological process, shaped by environment, culture, economics and politics. In recreating and debating their work over the past quarter century, the Witness Seminar participants – researchers, medical practitioners, midwives, industry representatives and breastfeeding activists – remind us of the very important questions that have and that continue to influence our study of health practices. The questions must and will be asked, though we recognize that the answers are always contingent and they more often than not give rise to still other questions. The testimonies at this Witness Seminar clearly demonstrate that despite all the studies on the physiology of maternal nursing, on the benefits of breast-milk and on the factors that inhibit and encourage mothers' nursing, breastfeeding is not an unquestioningly accepted part of the children's lives. But the drive to better understand the process of breastfeeding will and must persist if we are to ensure the health and well-being of future generations.

Rima D Apple
University of Wisconsin-Madison

THE RESURGENCE OF
BREASTFEEDING, 1975–2000

The transcript of a Witness Seminar held by the Wellcome Trust Centre
for the History of Medicine at UCL, London, on 24 April 2007

Edited by S M Crowther, L A Reynolds and E M Tansey

THE RESURGENCE OF
BREASTFEEDING, 1975–2000

Participants

Mr James Akre

Professor Elizabeth Alder

Mrs Phyll Buchanan

Professor Forrester Cockburn

Ms Rosie Dodds

Mrs Jill Dye

Professor Fiona Dykes

Ms Hilary English

Miss Chloe Fisher

Professor Anna Glasier

Professor Lars Hanson

Dr Elisabet Helsing

Dr Edmund Hey

Professor Peter Howie

Professor Alan McNeilly

Professor Kim Michaelsen

Mrs Rachel O'Leary

Ms Gabrielle Palmer

Professor Malcolm Peaker

Dr Ann Prentice

Professor Mary Renfrew

Mrs Patti Rundall

Ms Ellena Salariya

Dr Felicity Savage

Professor Roger Short

Dr Mary Smale

Dr Alison Spiro

Dr Penny Stanway

Dr Tilli Tansey

Mrs Jenny Warren

Professor Lawrence Weaver (chair)

Mr John Wells

Professor Brian Wharton

Professor Roger Whitehead

Dr Anthony Williams

Miss Carol Williams

Dr Michael Woolridge

Among those attending the meeting: Mrs Janette Allotey, Mrs Jane Britten, Ms Charlotte Faircloth, Ms Rachel Hillman, Ms Naomi Lewis, Dr Rhona McInnes, Professor John Walker-Smith

Apologies include: Professor Jaques Bindels, Professor Peter Elwood, Professor Stewart Forsyth, Professor Armond Goldman, Ms Sheila Kitzinger, Dr Penelope Leach, Professor Alan Lucas, Professor Pearay Ogra, Dr Andrew Radford, Dr Aileen Robertson, Professor Wendy Savage, Dr Andrew Stanway, Professor Daffyd Walters

Dr Tilli Tansey: I am the convenor of the History of Twentieth Century Medicine Group, which was started by the Wellcome Trust in 1990 to bring together medical historians, medical practitioners and others who have contributed to events in postwar medicine. Just over ten years ago we designed these Witness Seminars, to get people who have been involved in particular discoveries, debates or advances, to come and sit together in a chairman-led meeting to discuss what really happened, how things did happen, and why they happened the way they did.

The topics for these meetings are chosen by a programme committee of scientists, clinicians and historians. There are usually 20 or 30 topics suggested each year, and this topic was from Lawrence Weaver, who very kindly agreed to chair this meeting today. So without further ado, I will hand over to Lawrence to introduce the topic of the meeting and say something about the subject.

Professor Lawrence Weaver: Thank you everyone for coming. Breastfeeding may seem a rather obscure and arcane subject for a history of medicine Witness Seminar, but, of course, breastfeeding affects the early health, even survival, of babies and can protect them from disease in childhood and in later life. This Witness Seminar is devoted to what happened to breastfeeding over the last 30 years or so.

There seems to have been an upturn in the incidence of breastfeeding over the last 25 years, after a steady decline during the first half of the last century. During this period we have witnessed increasing concern about the declining numbers of mothers who wished to breastfeed their babies and efforts have been made to reverse this trend. This has brought together paediatricians, obstetricians, nutritional scientists, lactational physiologists, public health professionals, women's organizations, the church, pressure groups and international agencies in various combinations and alliances. These efforts have occurred against a background of the development and promotion of breast-milk substitutes. Infant formulae have become more refined to resemble human milk, are international in use and brand-led. A few big companies now control the supply of baby milks throughout the world.

Gathered here today are representatives of most of these groups and my hope is that we can explore this story, covering the period we have lived and worked through. I chose 1975 as a starting point because it represents a nadir in breastfeeding rates;[1] also, 1975 is about as far back as most of us can remember,

---

[1] See note 8.

or should I say as far back as we are likely to have been professionally involved. So, before we get going, I want to sketch out briefly how I think we reached what we now probably all agree is a very dismal situation, a state of affairs where the majority of mothers in this country, and also in parts of the US and elsewhere, never nursed their babies, had no intention of doing so and were given little support or help in suckling them, even if they had wished to do so. Bottle-feeding had become regarded as normal, not just socially, but also medically, and in the minds of some members of the medical profession, as better than the breast for mothers and babies.

Let us go back 100 years, to try to identify how such a state of affairs came about. Before the development of clean and nutritionally balanced human milk substitutes, not being breastfed during the early months of life was pretty much a death sentence. The Dublin Lying-in Hospital, for instance, in 1799 records a mortality rate of over 99 per cent in infants who were not suckled by their mothers.[2]

By the end of the nineteenth century, knowledge of the nutrient composition of human and cows' milk, an understanding of the energy needs of the newborn, along with recognition of the importance of clean milk with the introduction of sterilization, hygienic storage, etc., meant that bottle-feeding not only became possible, but saved lives. The growing employment of young women in the labour force and their social emancipation meant that many weaned their babies soon after birth. Feeding babies on artificial milk became a weapon in the battle to control infant mortality – then around 150 per thousand live births – and was given added urgency by the need to maintain a supply of fit young men for the imperial armies of Europe. Efforts to humanize bovine milk to mimic human milk brought together paediatricians, public health clinicians, chemists and food technologists.[3] Infant milk depots became a rallying initiative across Europe and North America and, although designed to promote and support breastfeeding, in many instances they became an outlet for modified cows' milk.[4] As a public health initiative, the depots largely

---

[2] Abt and Garrison wrote: 'Of the 10 272 infants admitted to the Dublin Foundling Hospital during 21 years (1775–96), only 45 survived, a mortality rate of 99.6 per cent' (1965): 81. See also Routh (1879): 243; Fildes (1985): 275, who quotes two earlier works, Forsyth (1911): note 39, and Wodsworth (1876): note 120.

[3] See Weaver (2006); Mepham (1993). For earlier accounts of the infant welfare movement, see Newman (1906); McCleary (1933).

[4] Ferguson et al. (2006); Weaver (2008).

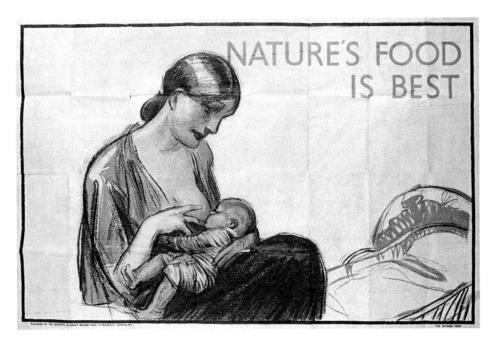

Figure 1: A mother breastfeeding her child, Lithograph, Wellcome Images.

disappeared by the end of the First World War, and by then dried milk had become widely available, formulae were on the market and the habit of bottle-feeding had caught hold.[5]

The acceptability and practice of bottle-feeding extended across the social classes, as it became regarded as safe, easy, convenient and affordable. The interwar years saw the start of a long, steady decline in breastfeeding, set in motion in part by the necessity of dealing with high infant mortality and poor infant health with safe formula feeding, among a raft of other maternal and child welfare initiatives.[6]

---

[5] Professor Lawrence Weaver wrote: 'The late nineteenth and early twentieth centuries saw the publication of many books about infant feeding, which had the effect of promoting infant formula. See, for instance, Cautley (1896); Cheadle (1889); Holt (1901); Dingwall-Fordyce (1908); Sadler (1909); Vincent (1910).' Note on draft transcript, 20 October 2008.

[6] Professor Lawrence Weaver wrote: 'These maternal and infant welfare initiatives included health visiting, maternity allowances, domestic science classes in schools and subsidized meals for young mothers. A number of historians have written about the relations between maternal and infant welfare, childbirth, infant feeding and efforts to control infant mortality. See, for instance, Apple (1986, 1987); Borst (1995); Dwork (1987a and b); Meckel (1990).' Note on draft transcript, 20 October 2008.

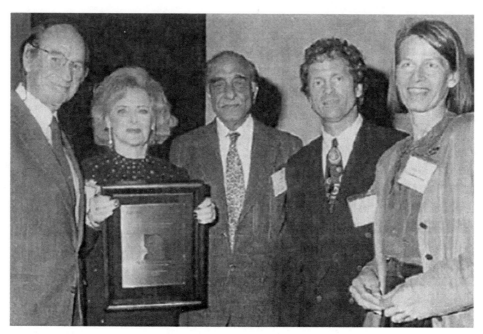

Figure 2: Professor E F Patrice Jelliffe at the Jelliffe Memorial Lecture, 1993, in memory of her late husband, Professor Derrick Jelliffe (1921–92), at the XVth International Congress of Nutrition Conference, Adelaide, Australia. L to R: Dr Michael Latham (presenter of the keynote address); Professor Jelliffe, Dr C Gopalan, Professor Irwin Shorr (chair) and Dr Elisabet Helsing. For further details, see www.waba.org.my/news/pat_jeliffe.htm (visited 20 January 2009).

By the 1960s a number of forces began to converge, or at least to excite the attention of those who cared for mothers and their babies. Paediatricians and nutritional scientists working in the developing world were not slow to appreciate the life-saving properties of human milk. Infant malnutrition stared them in the face and both public health initiatives and scientific research programmes began to focus on infant feeding. Derrick (Dick) and Patrice (Pat) Jelliffe's book, *Human Milk in the Modern World*, published in 1978, was both a powerful statement of the problem and a manifesto for action.[7] Paediatricians in the developed world were apparently too preoccupied with building up their subspecialties and even neonatologists had scant interest in how their patients were fed, especially after they had gone home. Obstetricians, in many cases, seemed primarily interested in safe childbirth from the mother's point of view and with it increasing hospitalization and medical control. Moreover, the dominant responsibility of midwives was to

---

[7] Jelliffe and Jelliffe (1978).

mothers and infant feeding seemed of little concern to them once the baby was delivered safely. Then the simplest thing to do was to provide formula with proper instructions on how to make up bottles and to leave mother and baby to get on with it. Even in maternity units, and particularly in the so-called premier units, such as the Simpson Memorial Maternity Pavilion in Edinburgh, breastfeeding rates in mothers leaving the postnatal wards dropped to below 20 per cent around 1970. I don't want to go into these figures in detail, but there is no doubt that the 1970s represent a nadir in breastfeeding rates.[8] Now this is a very broad-brush sketch of events and is designed simply to set the scene for our starting point in the mid-1970s. We may well pick up on some of these topics, even question my interpretation. One or two people here have queried the appropriateness of the term 'resurgence' of breastfeeding.[9] This is a fair comment and at the heart of the topics that I hope we will discuss. But, for whatever reason, it is a fact that breastfeeding rates were much lower in the 1970s than in the decades before, and lower than they are now. Perhaps the first question to ask is how we came to recognize that there was a problem. One answer to this must be the work done in the developing world and I am going to ask Roger Whitehead to set the ball rolling in that area.

Professor Roger Whitehead: Although historically it has not always been so, it is now widely accepted throughout the world that feeding a baby from the breast represents the best form of nourishment for the young baby and thus it is highly desirable. In the economically underprivileged populations of the world, however, it is something more than that, it is often a matter of life or death for the young child whether or not breastfeeding becomes established and is then continued for an appropriate length of time. The reason is well known to everyone here; there are no affordable alternative sources of food that come anywhere near to matching the complex nutritional needs of the infant. And this is compounded by the often impossible hygienic conditions that the mother has to face when she tries to make up such foods.

---

[8] See Table 1, page 9. Ms Rosie Dodds wrote: 'There may have been a nadir in 1975, but initiation rates in the UK remained almost completely unchanged as measured by successive Infant Feeding Surveys between 1980 and 2000, when rates started to increase in Scotland, so a resurgence in the UK is not evident [Bolling *et al.* (2007)]. In England and Wales, 67 per cent of mothers breastfed their babies at birth in 1980, 65 per cent in 1985 and 67 per cent in 2005, standardized for the age and educational level of women in 1985. The rapid decline in breastfeeding in the early days and weeks is also markedly similar across the decades.' E-mail to Ms Stefania Crowther, 9 December 2008. See discussion on pages 9–10.

[9] See pages 9–10, 65–6, 78–9; Appendix 2, page 89; and note 8.

Closely linked with this issue has been the historical debate about the length of time for which breastfeeding alone can satisfy the total nutritional needs of the growing baby. Largely on empirical grounds, a period of four to six months was suggested many years ago.[10] But this was not universally accepted by any means, not only by the food industry, of course, who had a vested interest, but, I am afraid, also by the paediatric and child health professions as well.[11] And, to compound this problem, when one measured the breast-milk intake of babies and compared these with the accepted energy requirements of young babies it indicated that the period for which exclusive breastfeeding was adequate was nearer to two to three months than four to six months. This was a scientific challenge my colleagues and I set out to investigate.

To cut a long story short, using both traditional and novel stable isotope techniques for measuring energy expenditure, we were able to show that between two and six months the energy requirements of such babies had previously been overestimated by as much as 25 per cent, and thus the average breast-milk intakes that we were measuring in these growing babies was actually sufficient for four to six months.[12] This work is, in fact, still being investigated via a multicentre study in Ann Prentice's department. We have to make absolutely certain that we have got everything right; it's such an important issue. I am confident, however, that what I have just said is much nearer to the truth than what was believed in the past.[13]

The energy requirements that I have just been talking about have, of course, now been revised by the World Health Organization (WHO) and the Food and Agricultural Organization (FAO). As part of this work that I have been discussing, we also thought it was important to re-investigate the growth of healthy young babies. We were able to demonstrate that the reference data for the growth of babies that had been used in the past were also misleading. The older growth reference data was indicating the beginnings of growth faltering and nutritional deficit in breastfed children much earlier than we now know

---

[10] See, for example, Hytten (1954).

[11] See Whitehead (1985).

[12] See Coward *et al.* (1979).

[13] Professor Roger Whitehead wrote: 'The final analysis from this large study has not yet been published but the results are compatible with what I have said.' Note on draft transcript, 30 November 2008.

Year	Unstandardized results (%)	Standardized for maternal age and education (%)
1975	50	
1980	67	
1985	65	65
1990	64	62
1995	68	62
2000	71	62
2005	77	67

Table 1: Percentage of mothers who began to breastfeed their infants, England and Wales.

Source: Bolling *et al.* (2007).

was correct.[14] I am pleased to say that the growth reference data have now been revised both nationally in the UK and internationally by the WHO.[15]

Weaver: Can we hear from the people with memories of actually what happened at the time – Brian, perhaps, or people who were working in the developing world – and how that might have impacted on what people were thinking about breastfeeding? That's a very helpful introduction, Roger, looking back to what happened, but can we get a feeling from the people who were on the ground?

Professor Brian Wharton: My comments wouldn't be about the developing world. If I stay just with the UK, we do have this very impressive set of national statistics collected by the Department of Health (DoH) and the Office of Population Censuses and Surveys (OPCS) and so on.[16] These showed that in 1975 about half of the mothers in England and Wales started off breastfeeding. The Simpson Memorial Maternity Pavilion must have been very unusual with 20 per cent. By 12 weeks, it was down to 15 per cent. Five years later, there was a quite definite change. When the 1980s arrived, about two-thirds of mothers started off breastfeeding. And at 12 weeks the 15 per cent had gone up to 27 per cent. So, there are some big changes in infant feeding between 1975 and 1980. The mysterious thing is that in the UK the trend seems to have stagnated, so, for example, if you take the figures for 2000, 71 per cent of women start off breastfeeding. So, you think, well, that's good, at least that's greater than 67 per cent. But the statisticians who write the OPCS report say that if you allow for such factors – that mothers are older now and better educated – overall, there

---

[14] Whitehead *et al.* (1981).

[15] WHO Multicentre Growth Reference Study Group (2006); Sachs *et al.* (2005); Dewey *et al.* (1995).

[16] DoH (2002); Bolling *et al.* (2007). The national survey has been conducted every five years since 1975.

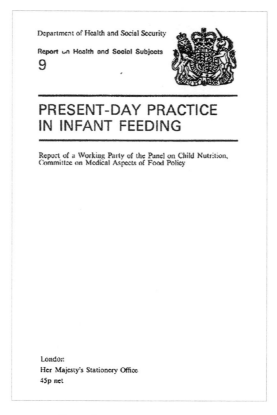

Department of Health and Social Security

Report on Health and Social Subjects

9

PRESENT-DAY PRACTICE IN INFANT FEEDING

Report of a Working Party of the Panel on Child Nutrition, Committee on Medical Aspects of Food Policy

London:
Her Majesty's Stationery Office
45p net

Figure 3: The Oppé Report, 1974.

has been no change.[17] So, that is historical fact. And it is well documented in national surveys.

The explanation: I don't know, and in particular why you get a substantial change from 1975 to 1980, and thereafter very little change. The evidence suggests there has only been a limited resurgence in the UK since 1980.[18]

Weaver: Was there any cross-talk, as it were, between what was happening in the developing world in the area that Roger Whitehead was talking about and your experience in the UK?

---

[17] See Table 1, page 9.

[18] Professor Brian Wharton wrote: 'There was a renaissance in the study of infant feeding, including breastfeeding, and an appreciation of its importance in the 1970s. The first "Oppé report" as it came to be known, was published in 1974 (Figure 3). There were subsequent reports with a similar title in 1980 and 1988 [DHSS (1980; 1988)].' Note on draft transcript, 31 August 2007. See also Glossary, page 128.

Wharton: I am not sure that there was in 1975. Everyone knew that it would be extremely dangerous not to breastfeed in the developing world. What was unusual was that an infant feeding report in 1974 said even in countries like Britain the desirable thing is to breastfeed your baby.[19] It doesn't sound like anything now, does it? But in 1974 it was comparatively revolutionary.

Dr Ann Prentice: You asked for a perspective on the developing world in the 1970s and the pressures in terms of policy with breastfeeding. At the time I started working in the MRC Gambia, with Professor Whitehead, in 1978, the prevailing idea there was that women living in underprivileged circumstances with a limited diet were not able to sustain an adequate lactational performance for more than about two to three months. So, combined with the ideas that we have heard from Professor Wharton and Professor Whitehead here in terms of the energy gap, these women were thought not to be able to produce milk of adequate quantity or quality.[20] I can remember attending a symposium with paediatricians in Mexico where we were told that the prevailing policy there was for health professionals to recommend women not to breastfeed if they had low intakes of particular micronutrients, calcium in this particular instance, and so women were being encouraged not to breastfeed or to wean their children at three months of age on to complementary foods, because of this concern about the gap.

As you know, infant growth faltering generally starts at around three to six months and it was thought to be very much tied in with the woman's ability to produce good-quality breast-milk. Back in the mid-1970s the World Bank was considering putting in place a number of feeding stations throughout Africa in order to provide extra food for lactating women precisely in order to improve their lactational performance, the quality of their milk and hence the growth of the children.[21] The work of the unit in the Gambia and elsewhere showed that in fact although that may have benefited the women to some extent – and that's no small benefit – the lactational performance of those women living in those circumstances, unless they were really on the edge of starvation, was actually very good. So the child itself was protected and there must have been other reasons for the growth faltering. In many ways I think that was the change in mindset that went on in the developing world at the end of the 1970s and

---

[19] Oppé *et al.* (1974).

[20] Whitehead *et al.* (1978; 1981).

[21] See Ronchi *et al.* (1976).

early 1980s in terms of the evidence that breastfeeding is best. Up until that point, the policy people out there, I think, felt that most of the women could not manage to breastfeed adequately for more than about two to three months. There was quite a revolution in thinking.

Weaver: So there wasn't any science before, and the sort of science that was being produced was slow to impact or have any effect on people? Was this new science, or a challenge to some sort of evidence-based thinking that existed before?

Prentice: I think a number of things came together at that time and part of it was new evidence about breast-milk volume using objective measures of milk intake rather than the culturally insensitive ways of trying to measure milk volume in the developing world that had been used up to then.[22] It was recognized that if you are analysing breast-milk for its quality you cannot use methods that are standard in the dairy industry, because it is not the same material.[23] There was a great push at that time to develop assay methods for looking at both the nutritional and the non-nutritional factors in breast-milk. And then there was the pioneering work on the antimicrobial properties of breast-milk, – Professor Hanson is sitting here next to me, I shall pass the microphone to him – the recognition that not only did breastfeeding protect in a passive way against infection, but also in a very positive and constructive way, and that these properties lasted longer than just during the colostral period. That was quite a different way of thinking about things back in the late 1970s and early 1980s.

Professor Lars Hanson: It is quite striking that we hadn't been aware of the capacity of previous generations to survive and this remarkable arrangement of the baby being delivered next to the anus of the mother to pick up the safest kinds of bacteria around, which quickly propagate, reaching high numbers; they cover the mucosal surfaces, especially in the gut, and keep away, or reduce the numbers of, more dangerous bugs to start with. Then the milk, which contains a very large number of protective components, protects against infection. But you could also say it protects growth by keeping the baby in such a state that it can utilize the nutrients provided by the milk, a much more refined and complicated system than we had previously understood. It is striking, for instance, that when we protect ourselves against infections, we almost always use mechanisms that induce inflammation. The inflammation results from a number of signals from

---

[22] Rowland *et al.* (1981); Coward *et al.* (1984).

[23] See Jensen and Neville (eds) (1985).

our host defence. But breastfeeding protects without inducing inflammation, a great advantage for the growing infant.

Weaver: Can you tell us about your personal experiences at the time and how you were led to take these views? I don't want you to theorize too much, I want to hear what happened.

Hanson: Well, you force me to tell you about my PhD thesis, which indicated that there was one major component in the milk, an antibody, which didn't look like other antibodies, and my thesis was accepted but the faculty said that this was biologically improbable. The story was, in fact, that this antibody, which was later labelled secretory IgA, makes up 80 per cent of all our antibodies. The reason that it is present in such a high amount is that it covers our mucosal membranes, and just the intestinal mucosa is about $400m^2$, so we need a lot because of that. The breastfed baby will receive as much as some 0.5–1 g per day of this protective component.

Weaver: So, this was a new and unique finding at the time. How was it received?

Hanson: It was received with quite some interest, especially after we found out that the secretory IgA antibodies in the milk were especially directed against the bacteria in the mother's gut. This makes a lot of sense because these bacteria are the ones the baby is normally colonized with after the normal exposure to them at delivery. The cells producing the secretory IgA antibodies migrate to the mother's mammary glands from special lymphocyte aggregates in her intestine, the Peyer's patches. Since the mother has been exposed to the microbes from her surroundings, the breastfed baby receives a very broad and efficient protection against microbes in its milk that otherwise could cause more or less severe infections in early life. This is likely to be an important protective mechanism and it has one aspect that is especially significant for the growing infant: in contrast to other defence mechanisms in the blood and tissues, it protects without causing an inflammatory response as most other defence mechanisms do. Inflammation has several negative effects on a growing individual, including decreased appetite.

Weaver: Did these findings impact on thinking outside of where you were working? How did they spread and did they affect thinking about breastfeeding elsewhere in Europe?

Hanson: Well, in a way it became the start of a series of studies from different places, showing that there are any number of components in the milk and some of them are working in very remarkable ways. One of them, lactoferrin, an iron-binding protein, is one of the major proteins of milk. Not only can it kill bacteria and viruses on its own, but it stops inflammation. Thus, it takes the risk of stopping this form of protective mechanism. This can take place because lactoferrin can, together with many other components in milk, defend anyway, and inflammation is the last thing the baby needs, because that inhibits growth by reducing appetite. The secretory IgA antibodies in milk are thus supported in this rather unique form of non-inflammatory host defence.

Whitehead: I will respond to one of your earlier points. One of the impacts, of course, was that we had to explain why the growth of even healthy babies appeared to be falling off at two to three months. If this really were true, then of course we would have to have a major rethink about weaning advice and weaning foods.

There is, however, another issue about the timing of weaning in the developing world apart from nutritional adequacy that was being thought about at the time. Even if the amount of milk produced by a mother in the developing world did not quite measure up to the complete nutritional needs of the child, it might be better to be left dietarily short rather than to try to introduce the potentially hazardous weaning foods that tend to be the only ones available in such economically deprived countries. This still remains a complex issue. There is a parallel with HIV-AIDS and advice for lactating women. Is it better for their babies to be breastfed, and thus risk the transmission of the HIV and a child dying of AIDS, or is it better that they be artificially fed and dyng from diarrhoeal disease if such feeds are not made up in a hygienic manner?[24]

Weaver: So the validity of existing dietary energy requirements was the origin of the 'energy gap' concept?

---

[24] Mrs Patti Rundall wrote: 'WHO held a technical consultation on HIV and infant feeding in Geneva in October 2006, updating its recommendations on infant feeding. A new UN consensus statement was adopted: "Exclusive breastfeeding is recommended for HIV-infected women for the first six months of life unless replacement feeding is acceptable, feasible, affordable, sustainable and safe for them and their infants before that time.... Breastfeeding mothers of infants and young children who are known to be HIV-infected should be strongly encouraged to continue breastfeeding.... Governments should ensure that the package of interventions referenced above, as well as the conditions described in current guidance, are available before any distribution of free commercial infant formula is considered."' Letter to Dr Daphne Christie, 3 September 2007. See www.who.int/child_adolescent_health/documents/ pdfs/who_hiv_infant_feeding_technical_consultation.pdf (visited 11 August 2008); Coovadia *et al.* (2007).

Whitehead: As I have said, the approach that we took was to find out, by scientific re-investigation of the whole issue of infant energy requirements, whether there really was an energy gap between requirement and what could be satisfied by breastfeeding around two to six months. Once we found out that previous estimates of energy requirements had been overestimated, the practical dietary advice became more straightforward. The advice that exclusive breastfeeding was normally adequate up to six months was correct.

In the late 1970s I had been a member of both Tom Oppé's Department of Health and Social Security (DHSS) Committee on Medical Aspects of Food and Nutrition Policy (COMA) committee on infant feeding as well as on the COMA committee that had been responsible for defining recommended dietary allowances (RDA) for energy, and it was a tremendous embarrassment to me when I realized that the two pieces of published advice were not mathematically compatible. That is one reason for our involvement. The main driving force for our 'energy gap' research, however, came from the developing world, where there clearly was a scientific problem of major importance to health education and child health planning that had to be faced.

Weaver: So this was really an indication of the 'weanlings dilemma', as it was then called, and the fact that there was no real definition of the optimum time to start weaning foods or to continue to breastfeed exclusively.[25]

Whitehead: Yes, we now know it is four to six months. The paediatrician Tom Oppé always said four to six months and Tom Oppé was correct.

Weaver: Based on what?

Whitehead: Professor Oppé's reasoning was mainly empirical, based upon clinical common-sense, I suppose that was what one would call it. But it didn't fit with the RDAs of that time and we scientists had to go back to the drawing board. By doing so we found out that we had been wrong.

Dr Edmund Hey: What we have already heard is that even today people are saying that growth falters at three or four months. They use a value-loaded word. What was really going on was that nobody had got growth standards, except Jim Tanner in this country and a few epidemiologists in the US.[26] These had been obtained, almost exclusively, from bottle-fed babies, so the whole world

---

[25] See Rowland (1986).

[26] Tanner *et al.* (1966a and b); Tanner and Whitehouse (1973): 787–8. See also Waterlow and Thomson (1979); Jelliffe and Jelliffe (1979); Waterlow *et al.* (1980); Whitehead and Paul (1984).

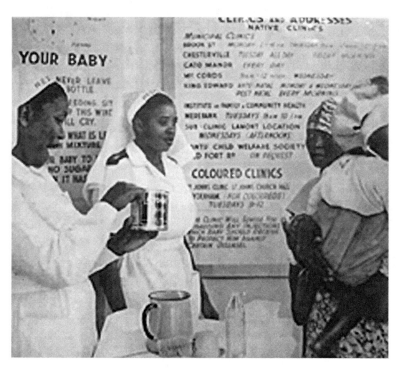

Figure 4: Nestlé Milk nurses in South Africa, c. 1950.

had become locked into what greedy bottle-fed babies will do when four or five months old; you push a little extra milk into them when they won't go to sleep.

Weaver: Was that truly the perception at the time? I think that is our perception now.

Hey: I was curious that people still use the word 'faltering'. It isn't faltering, it's a natural decline. The maximum rate at which a baby grows is at about 28 weeks' gestation *in utero*. At this time babies are growing at about 2 or 3 per cent a day, and this rate then gradually tails off, and they don't grow very much between one and two years. But there isn't a faltering, there is a natural decline.

Mrs Patti Rundall: I run Baby Milk Action and I only came into this work in 1980, but I just wanted to say that at that time Professor Whitehead's work was having a huge impact on people's understanding of the developing world, and we were extremely critical of it. Some of it was, I think, funded by the food industry, and we were concerned that this might have had an influence on the way the study was conducted and reported. The early research from the Gambia was certainly quoted by Nestlé and other companies at that time. It had a devastating impact on people's understanding. Nestlé used it to say that women could not breastfeed. They used it as an excuse, saying: 'That's why we have to do what we are doing; that's why we have to give free samples; that's why we have to do all these things.' So it was a huge problem for us.[27]

Weaver: Was the science thought to be suspect as well?

Rundall: Oh, absolutely. And I was very interested in what Ann was saying about the need to measure milk in a culturally sensitive way, which they did eventually. But I remember that in the early days the researchers did not measure the night feeding. So, this made us question how they could measure the volume of milk and what they meant by this 'faltering'. It was hugely controversial. Every time we put messages out that women could breastfeed, Nestlé would come back with a report from the Gambia proving that the companies were right.[28]

Weaver: I don't want to stop this discussion, but I notice that Dr Savage wants to say something. Are you going to stick with this topic?

Dr Felicity Savage: Absolutely. During this time I was working in Zambia and later on in Indonesia as a practical paediatrician, not a researcher, but growth monitoring of individual children was actively promoted. There was little concern with breastfeeding in either country. When babies were breastfeeding the growth tended to start decreasing from about the age of six months. A majority of babies grew very well for the first six months and then their weight gain would level off from about six months, with a clear cut-off time. Malnutrition in children under the age of six months mainly occurred when there was a real problem with breastfeeding and mothers were either mixed-feeding or were formula-feeding and not breastfeeding at all.

---

[27] Mrs Patti Rundall wrote: 'The later work that Ann Prentice refers to was hugely significant and much valued by the International Baby Food Action Network – the comments I made here related to the early Gambia studies.' Note on draft transcript, 3 September 2007.

[28] Mrs Patti Rundall wrote: 'This quotation from a *Guardian* article in 1990 gives an indication of the pressures faced by those managing research institutes who are often forced to accept funds from inappropriate sources: "The Director of the Dunn Nutrition Unit in Cambridge, Dr Roger Whitehead, has posted a notice to staff saying: 'At this moment in our fundraising programme, it is clearly important not to antagonize any part of the food industry unnecessarily. If you are asked by the press to comment adversely on a particular food product, can you please get in touch with me before proceeding.' Dr Whitehead said he did not wish to comment except to point out that the notice was a private message to senior colleagues, which only reinforced the policy of the Medical Research Council" [Erlichman (1990)].' Note on draft transcript, 3 September 2007.

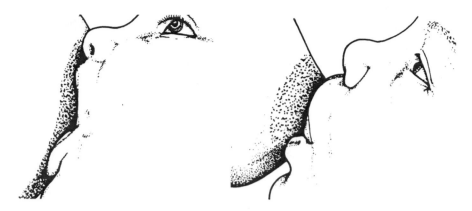

Figure 5: Good and poor attachment at the breast.
Left: Baby well attached, mouth widely open; lower lip everted; chin close to the breast.
Milk can be efficiently removed.
Right: Baby poorly attached, mouth not widely open; lower lip not everted; chin away from
the breast. Baby is sucking mainly on the nipple; milk is not efficiently removed, and the
nipple is likely to be traumatized.

In the population where I was working, mothers, when they had been breastfeeding for about three or four months, sometimes decided that they needed to go back to work, as their fields were getting neglected. They needed to start doing some farming. They would try leaving the baby behind, without breastfeeding during the day, so there were problems of growth then if they were fed on animal milk or formula, depending on what was locally available.

But another thing that we forget is that, at that time, people did not understand the management of breastfeeding. It was not appreciated that when a baby started to breastfeed, how the baby was attached to the breast and how frequently the baby fed, had a major impact on the production of milk.[29] It was always assumed if there was some concern about the quantity of milk that a mother might be producing, that this was due to her nutrition. Ann Prentice has already mentioned research that showed that this was not true. We really didn't understand the biology at that time.

Prentice: Three things: the first is to pick up again the points about growth faltering and absolutely accept the point that in terms of a healthy child with a well-nourished mother in good health care and so on, we now recognize that the pattern for the breastfed child is different from that of the child who is not breastfed. The new WHO growth charts show quite clearly that, even in the developing world

---

[29] See Figure 5, above, and Figure 10, page 61.

context, a child who is breastfed is likely to grow in the same way as if he had all the advantages of a child in the developed world.[30] So the growth faltering that I was referring to and that Professor Whitehead referred to earlier was actually the genuine growth faltering of children in the developing world who really do grow badly in the second part of infancy, a weight-for-age of around about -2 standard deviations (SDs) at one year, and height-for-age -1 SD. This is genuine growth faltering. That's what we were referring to.

Secondly, I don't particularly want to exercise the discussion with Patti we have been having for the last 25 years, but just to say that the work in the Gambia was never funded by the food industry and the work that we have been describing was an attempt to inject some objective measures into a debate that was definitely raging at the time about the type of data that was coming from the developing world.[31] There wasn't a recognition at that time of how inappropriate some of the methods that were being used were, as I said, either because they were not culturally sensitive – perhaps taking mothers away from their children during the night and so on, as you mentioned – or that they were using methods for analysing breast-milk which were not designed for human milk. And, I think, one of Professor Whitehead's legacies is his insistence on the real need to make sure that we used validated, objective measures for all the work that we did, and that has been seen with many other researchers as well, not just our group.[32] But that turned round a lot of the thinking, once we had some hard evidence that was not prejudiced by subjectivity, which many of the earlier studies had been.

And the final point was to introduce the way in which the ideas which were coming from the evidence from the developing world, which were designed to try to address the growth faltering of developing world children, then translated into the developed world. I started to see that happening in a number of ways. There was another look at the dietary reference values for this country in the

---

[30] Dr Ann Prentice wrote: 'The WHO growth charts can be accessed at www.who.int/childgrowth. These were obtained recently for children in different countries who were exclusively breastfed to six months. My comment about different patterns of growth between breastfed and non-breastfed babies cannot, therefore, be illustrated by providing a WHO growth chart. However, the history of growth charts and the differences in growth between breast and bottle-fed infants has been discussed in detail in a recent report by the Scientific Advisory Committee on Nutrition, *Application of the WHO growth standards in the UK*, available at www.sacn.gov.uk/reports_position_statements/reports/application_of_the_who_growth_standards_in_ the_uk.html (visited 19 February 2009).' Note on draft transcript, 27 October 2008.

[31] Prentice *et al.* (1980).

[32] See, for example, Whitehead and Prentice (eds) (1991).

late 1980s, when these concepts started to come through in terms of how one sets recommended dietary allowances for infants – 'reference nutrient intakes' as we call them now – and there was a recognition that we did not set one for breastfed children in the UK, in essence, and that for children who were not being breastfed, we did.[33] That was quite a change in thinking.

Another way that it impacted was in the way that women were supported to be able to breastfeed during their careers and, indeed, during the necessity of going out to work. I was very privileged to have been at a conference that was run at the Pontifical Academy of Sciences in Italy jointly with the Royal Society in this country. Professor Hanson was one of the organizers, so he could discuss that more, but at that time it was really to try to synthesize current understanding about lactational performance, about strictures, difficulties, limitations, barriers to breastfeeding from the mechanical – if you like, the biological – right the way through to the societal.[34] This was an attempt to try to introduce (in a policy way) through the Roman Catholic Church into areas like South America, the idea that women should breastfeed, that there was good evidence that women could breastfeed for three to six months or longer, and that it was good for the baby to be breastfed for that long, but that women needed to be supported. So, all of those things which came from the developing world to the transitional world and then into the developed world really started to change thinking.

Professor Mary Renfrew: I'm from the University of York. I wanted to reflect on how some of this discussion relates to my memories of being a student midwife in the Simpson and the Western General Hospital in Edinburgh in 1977. There are real resonances, because one of the things that people were starting to recognize at that time was a tremendous dissonance between what was coming from some of the scientific research, if you like, raising questions, undermining breastfeeding as an activity, and what some of the textbooks were telling us that we should be doing in terms of supporting the management of breastfeeding mothers, which was what it was called at that time. Therefore what we were being taught to do clinically was to measure, monitor, restrict and separate mothers and babies. That undermining message came both from the work we have been talking about just now, in terms of mothers' confidence in

---

[33] Hopkins *et al.* (2007).

[34] For the papers presented at the working group co-sponsored by the Pontifical Academy of Sciences and the Royal Society that met in Vatican City, 11–13 May 1995, see the United Nations University Press (1996), freely available at www.unu.edu/unupress/food/8f174e/8F174E00.htm#Contents (visited 11 August 2008). See also page 33.

breastfeeding and whether it was really enough, amplified by the undermining message coming from the medical and midwifery textbooks about measurement. As students we got this tremendous question: 'Would it work? Would it not?' This built a lack of confidence in breastfeeding that lots of people in this room have been trying to tackle ever since.

There were two things that I was conscious of as a student midwife. The first was that women's reports of breastfeeding were not in the literature. I went looking for them and, apart from Sheila Kitzinger's, accounts of what it was like to breastfeed in reality weren't there.[35] The second was the scientific evidence base around lactation: the quantity of milk women produced left to their own devices, when not monitored and measured and separated and so on. When I moved to Edinburgh, into a hugely privileged period of my life, with the people sitting in the row in front of me here,[36] we were trying to answer some of those questions. That was a huge step forward. But that dissonance between science and women's life experience and indeed the experience of some health professionals – and I am sitting beside Chloe Fisher, a major moving force, who kept reminding us that women really could do it, no matter what the scientists, medics and midwives tried to do – burgeoned in the late 1970s–early 1980s.

Weaver: May I bookmark that point and go back to finish with what was going on in the developing world? Maybe this is the moment for Lars Hanson to talk about lactation. But we will come back to midwife training, because I think that is the next big thing to concentrate on.

Hanson: I would like to ask a question. I think that we in the West have not doubted that the baby should be breastfed from the beginning. Why is it that so many traditional societies do not start at once? And this is a very dangerous thing to do, and you may have seen the beautiful report from Ghana by Karen Edmond and colleagues in *Pediatrics* just a few weeks ago, where she showed that starting breastfeeding within one hour decreased mortality by 22 per cent compared with starting on day three.[37] We have seen, for instance, that in Pakistan they give all kinds of things to the baby before breastfeeding starts one, two or three days later. Why is this very dangerous thing going on? It has gone on for a long time, or has it?

---

[35] Kitzinger (1962; 1980).

[36] Roger Short, Alan McNeilly, Anna Glasier and Peter Howie.

[37] Edmond *et al.* (2006) reported that 16 per cent of neonatal deaths could be prevented if all infants were breastfed from the first day and 22 per cent if breastfeeding started within the first hour after birth.

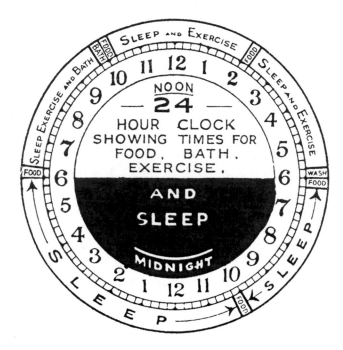

Figure 6: 24-hour clock, designed by Sir F Truby King (1913); reprinted 22 times up to 1932. Revised and reprinted in New Zealand 1937, reprinted twice to 1940.

Weaver: Were these ideas recognized at the time?

Hanson: I think this is very old, but I don't know, maybe somebody here can tell me. Why is breastfeeding starting so late and where did the idea come from? It is clearly very dangerous.

Ms Ellena Salariya: I'm from Dundee and I am, perhaps, the oldest person in the room, so I go back quite a bit. I do remember very clearly what was being advised regarding breastfeeding regimes when I began nurse training in 1950. Mothers were instructed to put their babies to the breast after six to eight hours if they were awake, as mothers were given sleeping pills routinely at this time. All babies, breast and bottle-fed, were given dextrose 5 per cent to test the patency of the oesophagus at four to six hours post-delivery. The few mothers who had chosen to breastfeed were screened off in the Nightingale ward and left to get on with it.[38] Midwives appeared to have lost interest in any skills in relation to this type of feeding.

---

[38] A Nightingale ward can accommodate up to 30 patients, with beds arranged in two long lines, 15 on each side, so that patients in the ward are all able to see one another, unless screens are used. See also page 64.

The mothers were advised, however, to 'time' the suckling and they all displayed their watches or clocks nearby; on the first day, one minute on both breasts was allowed at four-hourly intervals, this was increased to two minutes on day two, three minutes on day three and so on until ten minutes was allowed.[39] This prescribed time had been arrived at because a bottle-fed infant would consume formula milk from a bottle in 20 minutes.

I firmly believe that this is where many of our problems have stemmed from. The breastfed infants did lose up to 10 per cent of their birth-weights, not surprisingly, since they were being starved for several days after birth. This birth-weight loss is still accepted today despite several studies demonstrating that in the absence of early mismanagement of breastfeeding it is not normal that breastfed infants lose more than up to 6 per cent of their birthweight before beginning to regain the lost weight. Only this week I spoke with midwives at Ninewells Hospital, Dundee, and they told me that it is now considered normal for a breastfed infant to lose up to 11 per cent of his birthweight.

Weaver: So, this was the standard practice in teaching in maternity units and lying-in wards in the 1970s. Let's hear more about that.

Miss Chloe Fisher: This is modern: we move on to 1982, and this is a book written by Dr Miriam Stoppard, *A Complete Guide to Baby Care.*

> Introduce your breast gradually to the rigours of sucking. The first breastfeed should be no longer than one minute at each breast and the feed continued for this length of time throughout the first day. On the second day you can increase the length of the feed to two minutes on each breast, and on the third day to three minutes, so that by the end of the week your baby will be feeding for ten minutes at each breast.

I didn't know there were ten days in a week! But something that was never mentioned in all this horrible time was the 'pauses'. Babies pause when they feed. And my breakthrough as a domiciliary midwife was to say: 'But they didn't tell us what to do about the pauses: add a bit of extra time.' And, of course, the moment you start adding a bit of extra time you have broken down the barriers. I thought I would just amuse, or shock, you with that one. Ten days in a week!

---

[39] Miss Chloe Fisher wrote: 'A quote I can't help sending! "A clock is an essential piece of nursery furniture, and the baby should be 'fed' by it. If it is asleep it should be wakened; and if, in spite of thorough rousing, it refuses to suck, it should miss a meal." From a lecture given by Frederick Langmead in 1915, published in National Association for the Prevention of Infant Mortality (1915).' Note on draft transcript, 13 October 2008.

Savage: May I respond to the earlier question about the delay in starting to breastfeed? To my understanding this is old Brahminical and Galenical teaching that spread to some parts of the world and not to others.[40] There are some communities where mothers start breastfeeding straightaway, for example in much of Zambia; but in other countries, such as much of Indonesia, they delay, either because they think that the colostrum looks like pus and is unhealthy, or simply because there isn't any milk there, so there is no point in feeding the baby and they should give something else. Also, Valerie Fildes reported that in eighteenth-century Britain the delayed start was common, until Cadogan recommended that babies start to breastfeed within a few hours of delivery.[41] Newborn mortality decreased when this practice was introduced, but there was no accompanying decline in overall infant mortality, so it was apparent that something special had happened in the first month.

Dr Elisabet Helsing: I'm from Norway. This is also to answer Professor Hanson's question. In Norway, in olden times, there was a habit of giving the baby a ritual meal as an introduction to the world and to ensure ample food later in life. I believe the ritual was common around the world. I know that it happened in India, where honey and ghee and other things were given to the baby.

I also wanted to add to what others have been saying about the health workers' contributions to breastfeeding. There was a nine-country study performed by WHO in 1975–78, published in 1981, called *Contemporary Patterns of Breastfeeding*, which reported that the more mothers in all of these countries were in contact with their healthcare system, the less they breastfed. Now WHO never highlighted this very much, it was hidden on page 149 of the published report, but I think it is quite an important finding.[42]

Weaver: So when did WHO seriously start addressing these issues and what is the origin of the breastfeeding initiative?

Helsing: It was actually the Protein–Calorie Advisory Group of the United Nations System (PAG), which took up this issue in the early 1970s, and in

---

[40] See Wickes (1953); Cadogan (1748).

[41] Fildes (1985; 1998).

[42] WHO (1981a).

this way brought it into the auspicious body of the UN.[43] In 1974 the first World Health Assembly resolution on the issue of breastfeeding and the harmful promotion of infant formula was adopted, noting the general decline in breastfeeding in many parts of the world. There are people here who could give further detail on this.

Mr James Akre: I was at WHO from 1980 until 2004. Building on what Elisabet Helsing has just said, the first World Health Assembly resolution to use the word 'breastfeeding' was adopted in 1974[44] – to put that into historical perspective, the first World Health Assembly took place in 1948 – and the second was in 1978, and on both of these occasions there were general references made to the reduced rate of breastfeeding prevalence and duration, and then specific references to the impact of promotional activities and the inappropriate marketing distribution of breast-milk substitutes.[45] This in turn led to the landmark October 1979 meeting on infant and young child feeding, jointly organized by WHO and the United Nations Children's Fund (UNICEF). I will let Patti Rundall address this, but this was, in essence, the beginning of the International Baby Food Action Network (IBFAN), various activist groups have coalesced around what became IBFAN, since 1979/80.[46] The Baby-friendly Hospital Initiative was begun by WHO and UNICEF at a meeting of

---

[43] World Health Assembly, Fourteenth Plenary Meeting, 23 May, 1974. For a list of publications, see Sachs (ed.) (1975). The quarterly *Food and Nutrition Bulletin* (1978–) incorporates and continues the *PAG Bulletin* (1967–77) of the Protein–Calorie Advisory Group of the United Nations and is published by the International Nutrition Foundation for the United Nations university in collaboration with the United Nations system standing committee on nutrition (SCN).

[44] The 27th World Health Assembly passed resolution WHA27.43 on 'breastfeeding' in 1974, (WHO (1974).

[45] Mr James Akre wrote: 'The first occasion for WHO's senior policy-making organ, the World Health Assembly, to speak of breastfeeding occurred in 1974 when it noted "the general decline in breastfeeding in many parts of the world related to sociocultural and other factors, including the promotion of manufactured breast-milk substitutes." The Health Assembly urged "member countries to review sales promotion activities on baby foods and to introduce appropriate remedial measures, including advertisement codes and legislation where necessary" (WHO 1974). The issue was taken up again in 1978 when the World Health Assembly recommended that governments give priority to preventing malnutrition in infants and young children by supporting and promoting breastfeeding, taking legislative and social action to facilitate breastfeeding by working mothers, and "regulating inappropriate sales promotion of infant foods that can be used to replace breast-milk" (WHO 1978).' Note on draft transcript, 7 October 2008.

[46] See Allain (1981). For the background to the establishment of IBFAN, see www.ibfan.org/site2005/ Pages/article.php?art_id=34&iui=1(visited 8 January 2009).

the International Paediatric Association in Ankara, Turkey, in 1991. This was the brainchild of James Grant, who very directly put his stamp on it by taking a joint statement on breastfeeding and maternity services which was published in 1989 from the policy level and moving it right into the maternity wards and hospitals of the world and branding it with the name we know so well today.[47]

Ms Gabrielle Palmer: To encapsulate this history: Valerie Fildes' historical research shows that breast-milk was always seen as a good thing.[48] But the fact that it came out of women was the problem. Breastfeeding women weren't supposed to have sex, to be temperamental or red-headed; if they did any of these things their milk wouldn't be good. Also, Rima Apple, who has done splendid work, shows that the attitude was the same when doctors took over infant feeding in the US.[49] Chloe Fisher, who is here today, will know this quotation, 'it is better to have the vegetarian, nerveless cow,' than a woman who has temper tantrums, is weak, failing, or hasn't eaten well.[50]

Then there was a lot of money to be made by the blossoming paediatric profession in the US, which Rima Apple displays wonderfully.[51] The whole thing is that we know that women were told what to do and what was seen as the right thing, but actually we don't know to this day what women have done in private. Women – and I would include myself here – lie to health professionals, because we do what we think is best in the end anyway, if we have the confidence to do so.

---

[47] WHO/UNICEF (1989). See www.who.int/nutrition/topics/bfhi/en/index.html (visited 29 January 2009). The Baby-friendly Hospital Initiative, a worldwide programme of WHO and UNICEF, established in 1991, was followed in 1992 by the establishment of the UNICEF UK Baby Friendly Initiative, which was formally launched in 1994. See www.babyfriendly.org.uk/page.asp?page=11 (visited 17 June 2008), pages 43–5, 51–2, and Glossary, page 125. Dr Felicity Savage wrote: 'In the UK, from the beginning Professor David Baum wanted it to have a community component, so the word Hospital was dropped. It is hosted by UNICEF in the UK and is called the UNICEF UK Baby Friendly Initiative, which started in 1992. The importance of this is that it was considered important to make it a truly global programme, not just a programme for developing countries, because breastfeeding rates are lower in developed countries than in developing countries. However they are part of the same programme with the same aims and methods.' E-mail to Ms Stefania Crowther, 12 February 2009. For biographical information on James Grant see www.unicef.org/about/who/index_bio_grant.html (visited 13 October 2008).

[48] See, for example, Fildes (1998).

[49] Apple (1980; 1987).

[50] Ms Gabrielle Palmer wrote: 'Miss Chloe Fisher has often used this quotation from Dr Eric Pritchard, an early twentieth-century British paediatrician. [Pritchard (1907)]' Note on draft transcript, 3 September 2007.

[51] Apple (1994).

Historically, UNICEF and other international agencies so valued cows' milk as a wonder food that after the Second World War, they distributed milk on a large scale worldwide.[52] In non-milk-drinking societies, people naturally perceived this as a breast-milk substitute.

Weaver: The work of Valerie Fildes and Rima Apple belongs to the early part of the twentieth century. We want to concentrate on how we started going in a different direction.

Palmer: If I may come to this, please, those philosophies and ideas are still here today. People talk about 'the breastfeeding type', but there is no such woman. Industry exploits this very well. Infant formula is being distributed in Iraq now because the Iraqi people want it, because artificial feeding became established.[53] I loved it that Elisabet Helsing brought out the point that the more contact women have had with health workers the more breastfeeding has declined.[54] Maybe this is because we humans sabotage and compete with each other, even if it's subliminal. We talk about 'breastfeeding management' and that midwives are not interested, but in the past, infant feeding was something that women did that was part of the family culture. Now it is a medicalized, health-service-controlled matter. Women feel they need to read leaflets and ask a midwife, nurse or doctor to help them breastfeed. This mega-cultural change across the world has made women stop believing in their own bodies and this is a key factor.[55] I equate this lack of confidence with mass impotence in men. Maybe now we have Viagra my argument no longer works.

Weaver: I want to hear from these people who were actually involved in the maternity wards at the time. Roger Short, do you want to say something?

Professor Roger Short: Yes, if I could go back to the beginning and think about the natural history of breastfeeding, which is something that nobody's mentioned yet, the key feature. We are, after all, mammals and the definition

---

[52] See King and Ashworth (1987 a, b and c); Clark (1996).

[53] Ms Gabrielle Palmer wrote: 'Sources are Benyamin and Hassan (1998); personal communication from Dr Sami Shubber, former senior legal counsel at WHO Geneva, 1995; personal communication from Dr Naira Hasan, senior paediatrician, Baghdad Hospital, 1991; personal communication from Dr Yvonne Grellety, former nutrition in emergencies officer, 1999.' E-mail to Ms Stefania Crowther, 1 December 2008.

[54] See page 24.

[55] For Wendy Savage's comments about the over-medicalization of childbirth, see Christie and Tansey (eds) (2001b): 54–5.

of a mammal is that our young are exclusively, and I mean exclusively, fed with breast-milk for a varying period of time, depending on the mammal. So, what is the normal pattern of breastfeeding for humans? We have heard people talking about developing countries and developed countries, but, of course, they are all contaminated by western culture. When I was toying with the idea of leaving Edinburgh in 1982 and going to Australia, everyone said: 'Oh you are a silly idiot to leave Edinburgh, you like history so much, and if you go to Australia, it's all so new.' Somebody else said to me, 'But, of course, there's one thing about Australia, people have lived in Australia ten times as long as they have ever lived in the British Isles.' And I said: 'What?' I couldn't believe it.

When I arrived in Australia, I went to live with an Aboriginal group, the Jigalong mob up in the north-west of Western Australia, just to see a traditional human society that had only in the last couple of hundred years seen its first Europeans, and learn how they breastfed. It's an amazing experience and a vanishing one, but basically, as we had learnt from the studies of the !Kung hunter-gatherers in the Kalahari, surprise surprise, all women breastfeed, every single one; there isn't such a thing as a woman who can't breastfeed; it would mean she wasn't a mammal. What the Aboriginals and the !Kung hunter-gatherers do is put the baby to the breast immediately. It feeds for about one to two minutes per feed, four times an hour, throughout the day and the night. That's about 98 feeds per day and that is the normal pattern of breastfeeding for them.[56] I took on a very bright young American graduate from Harvard, Janet Rich, whom I put to live with an Aboriginal community (on Elcho Island) up in the Gulf of Carpentaria for a year and I said: 'There are about 100 mothers and babies there, and I would like you to study how they breastfeed. Let's ask one or two simple questions: how often in a day do you hear babies crying, and how often do you see a baby suck its thumb?' In one year, studying 100 children, she never once saw a thumb being sucked, it was always the breast, and you'd never hear a baby cry, because the nearest lactating mother would pick it up and feed it. Until we go back to the beginning and look at societies like the Australian Aboriginals, who have been in Australia for at least 45 000 years and only in contact with western society for 200 years, we will never know what normal breastfeeding represented. So I think we have got to go back to our beginnings if we really are to understand normal breastfeeding, and the horrific way in which we have abused it by giving the wrong advice down the centuries.

---

[56] Short (1992).

Weaver: So, did these sorts of ideas affect you, Mary Renfrew? You were saying that you were looking around for inspiration and guidance. Was it this sort of thinking that actually affected you at the time and answered your needs?

Renfrew: As a just-qualified midwife I didn't quite know what to do with myself, because I didn't like the health service that we ran, it didn't work for women. It didn't work for midwives, in my experience, either. And I was just phenomenally lucky because a job was advertised in the MRC reproductive biology unit, Queen's Medical Research Institute, Edinburgh (CRB), which Roger Short was directing at that time – working with Peter Howie and Alan McNeilly. I got the job and quite a lot of the rest is history, because we spent the next four years having immense fun doing a whole lot of studies which I am hoping Peter and Alan are going to talk about, in which I learned about why we should have confidence in breastfeeding physiologically, but also about the huge cultural limitations to it, which refers to what Roger has just said, and about women's real lived experiences, which others have talked about.

Professor Peter Howie: I was working in Glasgow when a job came up in Roger's unit, at the MRC reproductive biology unit in Edinburgh, and David Baird persuaded me that they needed a clinician to go through and, at a very alcoholic evening, I agreed. David sent me the five-year programme for the MRC unit and as I was very busy I hadn't had a chance to read it. I was going to see Roger, so I read it on the train journey between Glasgow and Edinburgh, which is 45 minutes. The first section included one statement that lactational amenorrhea protected against more pregnancies than all forms of artificial contraception put together.[57] I have to say that was the first time I had ever heard of the idea. I went into Roger and he asked: 'What are you interested in?' I replied: 'This lactational amenorrhea', and Roger said: 'Splendid, you are the man for the job'. He then sent me to see Alan McNeilly who had been researching the physiological basis of lactational amenorrhea, really trying to understand what happened when a baby suckled at the breast and the huge impact of neural impulses going to the brain hypothalamus and what actually happened thereafter. The MRC had been trying to understand that and now they wanted to see, using translational research, what impact that had in the clinical sphere. But before we talk about what we did clinically, we really have to start thinking about what the physiology was saying, because that was really the initial stimulus. Then I think that Roger wanted somebody like me to start

---

[57] Professor Peter Howie wrote: 'The document I referred to was an unpublished internal document of the MRC reproductive biology unit. See Buchanan (1975).' Letter to Mrs Lois Reynolds, 17 October 2008.

to help looking at what was happening to patients. So it was the physiological understanding that was being explored first.

Weaver: And what year was this famous train journey?

Howie: 1978.

Professor Alan McNeilly: It was one of the best days of my life, Christmas 1975, when Roger Short offered me a job at the MRC centre for reproductive biology and I am still there. I should have kept the telegram that came to Winnipeg offering me the job when I was on sabbatical, having been at Bart's Hospital, London, working on prolactin, which had only been discovered about four years before, around 1971. People thought it was a growth hormone, because all the bioassays that we used were animal bioassays, and human growth hormone promotes lactation in animals, but doesn't in humans. The whole purification process was skewed by that. People didn't even know that human prolactin existed. There was a huge myth until about 1972 that humans were different anyway.[58] That was a starting point, because Roger had identified the concept that the number of births that were prevented just by breastfeeding was far exceeding anything until oral contraceptives came in. I had done some work with Roger with his PhD student Ken McNatty, and we are still working together now, on the effects of prolactin on the ovary. I went to Canada from Bart's and was recruited back to Roger's unit in 1976. My first degree is in agricultural science, and so is my second degree, and then I ended up at Bart's Hospital having to learn clinical endocrinology.

The reason I am telling you this is because when I was then asked by Roger Short to investigate lactation and fertility, I was absolutely amazed at the ignorance of the clinicians who were dealing with this. They had absolutely no idea how lactation worked, even the basics of oxytocin release for milk ejection. Well, of course, when the baby is born, to get the placenta out you give oxytocin (Syntocinon), but actually the baby suckling releases oxytocin, it's the natural way to deliver the placenta. If you don't do that, well, there will be problems. But besides that, the whole concept of suppressed fertility in lactation was considered a bit of a myth really, wasn't it Roger?

People did not believe it, because they breastfed once a day and their menstrual periods would come back. So, we had tried initially with an MD student, Christine West, to get access to patients to actually track what was going on.

---

[58] See Forsyth (1970); Bonnar *et al.* (1975); Short (1976).

At that time endocrinology was: we have a compound, we will inject it and see what the compound generates. We inject gonadotropin-releasing hormone, see how much hormone is coming out of the pituitary gland and we will relate that to the onset of menses. The problem was that it was cross-sectional; we planned to take 100 women, inject it and measure it at three months and six months and try to understand what was happening. It was completely hopeless, but to try to get any studies done in Edinburgh, or anywhere actually, tracking normal women was almost impossible as well, because the will wasn't there. I was going to say because it wasn't a conceived idea, but it just wasn't on the radar. When Peter arrived, we gelled immediately and I told him that we needed to track normal women through their lactation. Roger had suggested it and then we could do it.

We did a simple thing. We got our breastfeeding women to collect urine specimens once a week. David Baird was the inspiration for this.[59] This is how he tracked infertility patients. We would do the same thing. Once a month we would go back and collect the samples. They put the samples in the freezer. Christine West and I had done an initial study to see how long women would breastfeed.[60] Well, they breastfed for two months. Peter and I worked out that we needed 120 women, I think, to actually get statistically meaningful data. We also did something which you shouldn't do, we gave them a calendar on which we asked them to record when they breastfed and for how long; what menstrual periods they had; anything like this. It had never been done before. So, we had real data from real women in real time and could relate these to the resumption of menstruation with all these patterns. This was an amazing difference, because it was, I think, the first-ever study of this kind that actually showed that infertility did happen, that fertility was suppressed by breastfeeding. It was very, very clear; it was unambiguous; you could not dispute it any more. But, people still did.

Weaver: What connection or reference was there to the developing world, where this was common practice? People must have observed this to be the case there.

McNeilly: My recollection – Roger can fill in better on this – is that the data was so poor, so bad, that there was no point even looking at it, because it was all cross-sectional, there was no tracking data. The problem that the effects on fertility vary between women was the big thing that we came across. Peter

---

[59] Baird (1979).

[60] West and McNeilly (1979).

Howie could expand on this. I remember one day in the coffee room in the old MRC centre for reproductive biology in Edinburgh we had a blinding flash of inspiration related to supplementary food and the effect it had, and how the system was actually working.

Howie: Yes, in fact we didn't need 100 women, because the effect was so obvious that when the women were suckling regularly without supplementary food, they all suppressed all ovarian activity and did not menstruate. And it was just abundantly clear that when supplementary food was introduced to the babies it immediately signalled a reduction in the number of times mothers would suckle their babies every day, and that was the point at which you started to see some ovarian activity taking place. Some of the cycles were not normal, there were inadequate luteal phases, but when ovarian activity started, you could have break-through ovulation and the risk of pregnancy. So, the key point that came out was that it's the amount of suckling that actually controls the amenorrhea and the infertility. The early introduction of supplementary food, which we have heard about for nutritional reasons, was undoubtedly undermining the effect of lactational amenorrhea, shortening the birth intervals and all the social consequences that that led to. As a result of the understanding of the physiology and the clear demonstration of what was happening biologically, there then emerged a number of initiatives looking at the impact of feeding patterns on birth spacing in developing world countries. Particularly the Bellagio Consensus, which emerged as a very important event, with guidelines about the amount of feeding that you require to maintain a very high chance of suppressing ovulation.[61] And also, WHO did a seven-country study that showed that the suppression was true in whatever country, be it developing world, intermediate world, or developed world. It was true across all cultures that if the mothers suckled often enough, they suppressed ovulation. And the response to all this was to get messages out that birth spacing through breastfeeding was still a very important part of managing fertility control.

Weaver: I know Lars Hanson has an interest in this and was instrumental in it affecting the thinking of the Catholic Church.

Hanson: It became very obvious in the 1970s and 1980s that the very high infant mortality was closely related in poor parts of the world to high fertility. And it was realized that reducing fertility to a spacing of more than two years reduced infant mortality by 50 per cent. So it would be extremely important

---

[61] Family Health International (1988). See also Short *et al.* (1991); and Glossary, page 125.

to spread information about this effect of promotion of breastfeeding and I felt that the Pontifical Academy of Sciences would have the power to provide this very broad message, getting around the fact that they, for religious reasons, could not propagate other forms of hindrance of fertility. It took a very long time, it actually took several years until it became possible to arrange the meeting that Ann Prentice referred to.[62] Actually a report resulted from the Academy that supported this aim of ours, and I can't tell you how efficient it was, but at least it became an issue, also, for the Catholic Church.[63]

Weaver: And you met the Pope?

Hanson: Oh yes, that was part of it. Twice, actually.

McNeilly: Just one thing about the 120 women that we started with in the Edinburgh study. Because of a certain Mary Renfrew who actually collected the data, we reviewed the data after six months and we had only got data-complete sets on about 20. We couldn't understand this, and, of course, what was happening was that Mary was acting as the buffer for problems that the mothers were having during breastfeeding. She was being able to mentor them through the problems. Also the diary sheet of each woman was very interesting, because we found all sorts of things about their family lives, what they bought at Safeway, what they didn't, the problems with the cars and everything like that, and the life history of these women was on this documentation, which was really important.

---

[62] See discussion on page 20.

[63] Professor Lars Hanson wrote: 'I tried many channels to approach the Pope including through the Archbishop of Vienna, and the vicar in the Pope's own parish in Rome. Finally this resulted in an invitation to a study week on resources and population at the Pontifical Academy of Sciences in the Vatican in 1991. I was to be given the opportunity to present my case in ten minutes under the chairmanship of Professor John C Waterlow. However, he fell ill the evening before this session was to take place and I was asked if I could replace his lecture and give a 45-minute presentation about the role of breastfeeding in controlling population growth and decreasing infant mortality. I did so using especially the data from our work in Pakistan and Central America illustrating the problems with the rapid population increase coupled with high infant mortality and often limited breastfeeding. A very intense discussion followed. During the study week we met His Holiness Pope John Paul II…. However, nothing much happened after this, so I continued to try to have the Vatican and its Pontifical Academy of Science act more efficiently in spreading the message that breastfeeding could make a big difference in areas with much poverty, fast population growth and limited breastfeeding. Ultimately there came about the renewed meeting at the Vatican's Academy of Science, which I attended in the company of Ann Prentice and Peter Howie. During that meeting we did produce a statement supporting the use of breastfeeding for all its good effects. I believe that statement was widely distributed, but I do not know how effective it was.' Note on draft transcript, 12 September 2007. See Pontifical Academy of Science working group (1994; 1995); Pope John Paul II (1995).

And it was such a simple thing, because it was an A4 sheet of paper; that's all it was; but we had there, documented, what really happened in their lives in relation to those potential factors that affect fertility. Several things came out of this, but I remember one of the key things was that we never actually achieved the total number of 120 women. I think all the data we collected over the years was from about 70 women all the way through, and then Anna Glasier joined us and we did more intensive studies. Nevertheless, it was because the mothers had somebody who knew what to do, how to fix the problems, and they knew she would come to collect the samples and to talk to them. It made an enormous difference. It could, of course, have screwed up the whole study, because if we had needed 120, we would never actually have published anything.

Tansey: May I ask you where the data sheets are?

McNeilly: They are probably in a box in one of our animal houses, because that's the safest place to store them.[64]

Professor Anna Glasier: To take the story of the work that we were doing on the resumption of fertility postpartum a little further. After Alan, Mary and Peter started to publish the initial studies in Edinburgh, I, as an evil doctor who knew absolutely nothing about the physiology of breastfeeding, was then recruited to look in more detail at the hormonal changes underlying lactation and fertility. I then became a member of the natural methods task force of the human reproduction programme of the World Health Organization, and, of course, breastfeeding is a natural method of contraception.

And so in that context we really did two things at WHO – *they* really did two things at WHO, I was very peripheral to it – we set up a huge seven-country study of over 4 000 women followed from childbirth until they had had two normal menstrual periods – which for many of them was 18 months or so later – looking at patterns of breastfeeding and the resumption of fertility postpartum.[65] This confirmed the findings that had been published from Edinburgh, that the resumption of fertility depended on how enthusiastically, how often, you breastfed your baby, and when you introduced supplementary feeds.[66] At the

---

[64] Professor Alan McNeilly wrote: 'At present, our searches for any of these forms have been unsuccessful. The studies are now all more than ten years old and past the time that we are obliged to keep such documentation. We do not have storage space for all the paperwork to be kept after this time and so any may have been shredded.' E-mail to Mrs Lois Reynolds, 13 August 2008.

[65] See WHO Task Force on Methods for the Natural Regulation of Fertility (1998a and b; 1999a and b).

[66] Howie *et al.* (1981).

same time that we were doing this study, the human reproduction programme (HRP) and others, and particularly a group working in Chile with Horatio Croxatto, a scientist at the Catholic University in Chile, and some people in Washington DC who were interested in natural family planning methods, attempted to turn breastfeeding into a kind of official method of contraception by calling it the lactation amenorrhea method or LAM. That was really born at another Bellagio Consensus conference and LAM is still a recognized formal method of contraception in all WHO's current publications on guidelines on contraceptive use, LAM features as a method of contraception.[67] And much of the work that was done in the mid- to late 1980s, again often in Chile, to prove the effectiveness of LAM has really never developed any further. LAM is there, but I think all research on LAM really stopped in the early 1990s when the proponents moved on to other things like emergency contraception.

Weaver: Who sponsored the Bellagio meeting? Was it WHO that initiated it?

Short: I was on the HRP as an adviser to WHO from 1972 to about 1985, I think, and we got breastfeeding steered through as one of the priority areas for the HRP study. The Director General of WHO – and Jim Akre will bear me out on this – was Dr Halfdan Mahler, and I remember Mahler saying to me: 'You know, WHO made a big mistake. We came out with these recommendations about the marketing of breast-milk substitutes but we didn't first come out with a statement about the advantages of breastfeeding.' So it seemed very illogical, here was WHO taking a position against infant formula without ever having made the case as to why breastfeeding was better. And Mahler said that this was one of the things that he would always regret, that WHO had made a policy mistake in the order of its pronouncements.

But if I could just go back a moment, since we have raised the topic of fertility. Another example that came to us – and Mary, Peter, Alan and Anna will remember this clearly – was that we had a young Australian paediatrician working with us in Edinburgh, John Cox, who had been working up in the north of Australia and had carried out an amazing study of one Aboriginal woman – and I have her photograph with me today – who by the age of 20 had six children (Figure 7).[68] The reason for this was that the Premier of the state of Queensland, where she lived, had issued an edict that breastfeeding was primitive and all Aboriginal women

---

[67] Family Health International (1988); Kennedy *et al.* (1989). See also Short *et al.* (1991); Finger (1996); Labbok *et al.* (1997); Heinig (1998); Anon. (1988).

[68] Cox (1978).

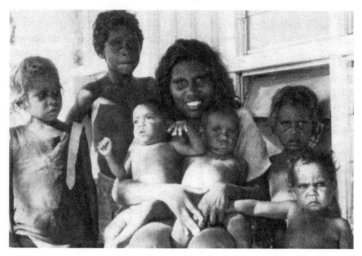

Figure 7: Aboriginal mother, aged 20 years, with her six children. Cox (1978).

should come into hospital to have their babies and should feed them on infant formula. John was able to document the birth weights, growth rates, moment of introduction of supplements and subsequent reproductive activity of this woman until the age of 20, by which time she had six children. That caused such a scandal that it actually reached the ears of the Governor-General of Australia, who changed Australian laws about what should be said to traditional Aboriginal women, and that to force infant formula on them was an absolute disaster. So we did actually change the practice, and although Australian Aboriginal women are still severely disadvantaged, at least things are better than they were.

Dr Michael Woolridge: I wanted to add a date stamp to something that you were talking about earlier. I became a researcher in this area, I am surprised to hear, at about the same time as Peter Howie, about late 1978. A year earlier, in July 1977, our first child was born in Canada, and when we went to the bookshops to look for books on how to breastfeed, on breastfeeding management, there was only one single book on the shelves, and that was a fairly new Penguin book by Sheila Kippley, entitled *Breastfeeding and Natural Child Spacing*, so quite clearly there was a current of belief, although it hadn't yet been adequately researched, that a commitment to breastfeeding would establish effective natural child spacing.[69] The adverse effect of this for us was that as I was a trained zoologist in quantitative research methods and Sheila Kippley's book said the baby must be fed for ten minutes on both breasts, every two hours, I would be there with a

---

[69] Kippley (1973).

stopwatch in the middle of the night, and if our baby came off after six minutes I would try to encourage my wife to put her back on for another three or four minutes. A year later I became a researcher in the area!

Professor Elizabeth Alder: I joined the MRC reproductive biology unit in Edinburgh in the mid-1970s and was inspired by both Roger Whitehead and Alan McNeilly, and then Peter Howie and Anna Glasier. I am a psychologist and what was quite novel and one of the strengths of the unit was this multidisciplinary team. I was also a lactating mother and at the time I had breastfed three children. So I was aware of what was going on, and remember that the resurgence of breastfeeding was very much class-related; it was education-related, so my peers were beginning to breastfeed and I was happy breastfeeding. But I was also hearing on the unit that there was a fear, even then in the 1970s, of having fat children, and that breastfed babies would not be fat, and I don't know whether this is true or not, but that was the fear. This nutritional debate that bottle-fed babies would be overfed was the incentive to breastfeed babies, because there was a belief that you could not overfeed breastfed babies. That was a great incentive. How that ties up with nutrition overseas I am not quite sure, but it's interesting.

The other is the aspect of the timing. I think earlier on, as Chloe said, 'a minute or two each side.' I tried with the first child, after that with the other children, not at all. Mothers simply ignored it. The third thing is the lactational amenorrhea. I came trotting back to all my friends saying: 'Don't worry, if you breastfeed for 20 minutes and so many times a day, you won't conceive.' They would not believe it. We are so much a pill generation, so dependent on reliable contraception, that I don't believe that one of my contemporaries would have trusted lactation amenorrhea. Remember too that the lifestyle that people have, trying to get a baby to sleep through the night, not having them next to you in your bed, was not the same as in the developing countries. So, the influences that were coming from this kind of research weren't necessarily having an impact on mothers. I think it takes a long time to percolate down, and I think we should try to remember this communication between research and what's going on in real life.

Mrs Rachel O'Leary: I would like to mention a subculture that was going on at the same time. I was working as a breastfeeding mother in 1977 and in 1980 I was accredited as a La Leche League leader. By that time we had published our book *The Womanly Art of Breastfeeding*, which was the one that told you how to breastfeed, written from mothers' own experiences.[70] Of course, it was imported from the US, but we could handle that. It also told about suppressing periods and how you might even not conceive. That was something that was mentioned in that very old first edition of the book. It has been in print continuously since then and you can get the seventh edition nowadays. But the culture being built up was very much in spite of the health professionals. There was an air of excitement at those early meetings where we would all cram into somebody's front room and hear: 'Yes, it's really OK to feed the baby as often as you want. Yes it's OK, people do sleep with their babies, babies are allowed to feed at night.' All of these odd ideas were coming out, and we looked at each other and thought: 'Is it really true? Can we really do this? That woman over there, she does it.' It was really quite an amazing experience to be part of at that time. I have to say it's not that different now. We are still finding health professionals who are very hard to convince that breastfeeding is really any different from formula feeding, but nowadays we have a huge group of breastfeeding-aware scientists and health professionals who are a huge help. In fact, throughout those years there have been health professionals who have been terrifically helpful and given us advice and inspiration. Well, starting with the Jelliffes.[71] We had the Jelliffes' book in our La Leche League group library in 1977, and reading that opened people's eyes because we wanted to breastfeed because we liked it, it was convenient and we thought it was probably better for the baby's health. Seeing that babies were actually dying because they were not being breastfed and hearing experiences from developing world settings gave us fire in our bellies, which inspired us to help each other and to continue that support for other breastfeeding mothers, which is still really important.

Professor Malcolm Peaker: Speaking of the slightly developing world, but 1975 is pretty recent as far as I am concerned, because I started work on the mammary gland in 1968 and that seems a lot longer ago than 1975. The interesting thing was – and picking up on Alan's point, one of the great problems with working on the mammary gland in lactation – that all the previous work had been done in dairy animals, a blessing for endocrinology, but an absolute curse for physiology. The great problem was that the analyses were done in dairy terms by dairy chemists. They were the British Standards, and it was solids that were measured, not fat, ash, etc., which had no physiological conceptual basis whatsoever for any species. Like Ann was saying, there was a great problem in devising analyses not only for human

---

[70] La Leche League International (1963).

[71] Jelliffe and Jelliffe (1978).

milk but for all milks. The traditional dairy chemist would not believe that we could analyse 2 ml of milk and get all the information that we actually needed; they would take a few litres. The other great problem was that dairy scientists analyse bulk milk as you collect at the end of the milking from the entire period. People took spot samples from wild animals, from zoo animals, from women, and thought that represented the whole of the milk in that volume in the breast. Now, that is certainly true in some species, but in most it is not, because of the rise in fat from the alveoli milk. So there were these huge problems to overcome. At the same time we had to explain all those dairy science findings in exocrine-secretion terms. And we, Jim Linzell and I, really started – at Babraham Agricultural Research Council Institute of Animal Physiology, Babraham, Cambridge – to get the mammary gland recognized as an exocrine gland when the whole of physiology, if they worked on glands at all, used salivary glands, which either switch on or off, whereas the mammary gland, of course, secretes continuously when it is actually switched on but at a very low rate (1–2 g per g of mammary tissue per day).

It is physiologically so boring that, after I had worked on the salt gland for my PhD, I thought: 'I will never stand working on this, it takes you days to get data. It is five minutes for an experiment on the salt gland, wonderful.' And so all this exocrinology followed and it needed a new exocrinology because the mammary gland is unusual in that it stores its secretion between what the dairy scientists would call 'let-downs', but what Alan would now call 'ejections'. This also created the problem because, of course, it was thought that it was perfectly natural to leave milk to accumulate to measure the secretory rate and things like that, whereas, of course, in most species you can't actually let milk accumulate, it switches off in different periods. So that's why many of the milk secretory rates – in women, rats, mice and in pretty well anything you could mention – were wrong. Actually, a lot of the published data from the 1950s, 1960s and 1970s defy all logic, because the growth rate of the young is higher than the presumed secretory rate of every milk constituent.[72] So, essentially, everything had to be started from scratch to try to get this on track as a piece of exocrinology to go alongside the endocrinology that was going on, and then to link the systemic changes in the hormonal environment to the tactical control of secretion, the minute-to-minute, hour-to-hour secretory rates, which Peter Hartmann then picked up in Australia, to determine the secretory rate in the shortest possible period by computer imaging the breast in lactating women.[73]

---

[72] Linzell (1972).

[73] Daly *et al.* (1992).

Weaver: How was the link made between the animal physiology and human lactation?

Peaker: Initially by Mavis Gunther, would you believe?[74] She talked to Alfred Cowie at the National Institute for Research in Dairying, Shinfield near Reading, and then came to talk to us, saying: 'All these people are poisoning all the infants in Britain by making up milk too strong. You know something about osmolality and tonicity and things, don't you?' So I then ended up getting interested in human milk and the comparison with milk formulae. Then, of course, that interest spread on to other aspects like lactogenesis, and my wife does wish me to point out that her milk appeared in *Nature* in 1975, on the lactogenesis story.[75] My third son says it was milk that was intended for him and he has suffered as a consequence. But it was Mavis Gunther who was actually trying to make the links because she was totally frustrated, on the clinical side, that people weren't actually taking any notice from the human medicine point of view.

Renfrew: Thank you; that contribution has brought a number of names to mind that were terribly influential for me once we started thinking about the breastfeeding physiology studies that we went on to do. One is Frank Hytten, whose physiological studies were incredibly important;[76] Harold Waller, whose clinical studies were very influential, certainly to my thinking;[77] and Mavis Gunther, who has already been mentioned. But those three people gave us a real headstart, and, for me, Mavis Gunther still stands head and shoulders above most people in terms of her drawing out and describing the kinds of symptoms of breastfeeding when there are problems and what to do about them. And she really looked in great depth at nipple pain, bless her, in a way that very few people have done, which was incredibly helpful.[78]

Weaver: How did her work become well known?

---

[74] See Gunther (1963; 1975). See also pages 41, 51 and 56.

[75] Peaker and Linzell (1975).

[76] A series of 11 articles by Frank Hytten on 'Clinical and Chemical Studies in Human Lactation' appeared in the *British Medical Journal* between 23 January and 18 December 1954. See, for example, Hytten (1954). See also Thomson *et al.* (1970). Additional biographical and bibliographical information on Frank Hytten has been provided by Dr Edmund Hey and will be deposited along with other records of this meeting in archives and manuscripts, Wellcome Library, London, in GC/253.

[77] Waller (1952).

[78] Gunther (1953).

Renfrew: I am not sure that it did become well known. It was a well-kept secret. There's a Penguin book that was really hard to get but was given to me by Christine West, whom Alan mentioned. When I started working at the MRC reproductive biology unit in 1982, she said: 'Read this.'[79] It was actually quite difficult to get hold of for a while. She became influential to some of us, and to Maureen Minchin, indeed, who wrote *Breastfeeding Matters*, and was influential in another way, internationally.[80] Mavis Gunther inspired other people.

McNeilly: Related to what Malcolm Peaker was talking about and the dairy industry and using cattle as a basis of research: they store milk in a big cistern, the udder. As I had been milking cows, I knew that they would eject milk quite happily as they walked along and it wasn't difficult to get milk out of a cow's mammary gland. But women don't store it in the same way. It's stored in the alveoli and they need oxytocin to release milk. If they don't have oxytocin released then they actually have trouble getting milk to the baby. If you watch babies suckle, it's quite clear when the milk ejection does occur and they get a lot of milk. This is normal biology. This is physiology, and the person who did a lot of work on this, Dennis Lincoln, had shown in rats that in fact it was the mother's brain that released the oxytocin and made the baby suckle.[81] And one study that we did in Edinburgh is related to this; we showed that the baby crying would release oxytocin before the baby got to the breast.[82] A completely different system from what was in the textbooks then, and is still in the books, and is still wrong in lots of the books. In parallel with Malcolm, my wife and I – in an article published in the *BMJ* – showed milk ejection at absolutely precise intervals during lactation in a mother who suckled twins, who happened to be my wife.[83] This was 1978, and yet this whole story is not out there either, but one of the key things to this is that oxytocin is turned off by stress. If you stress somebody, you turn the oxytocin off, you can cause problems and it's a downward spiral. It doesn't matter how many times you say this to people, they chant: 'This is just physiology, so what's that got to do with people?'

Mrs Jenny Warren: I was the National Breastfeeding Adviser for Scotland, now very happily retired. I want to pick up when you mentioned Mavis

---

[79] Gunther (1970).

[80] Minchin (1989).

[81] Wakerley and Lincoln (1971); Lincoln and Paisley (1982).

[82] McNeilly *et al.* (1983).

[83] McNeilly and McNeilly (1978).

Gunther. There are a lot of wonderful people at this meeting who have been involved in research into lactation and associated aspects for many years. Early in that time I was a young midwife and had no clue about breastfeeding, but was lucky enough to come into contact with the National Childbirth Trust. The voluntary organizations to do with childbirth and lactation were very much working with mothers, and they then began to get together with the midwives, because there was a lot of medical intervention in childbirth and I think that was a very important time, bringing the health professionals, the mothers and the voluntary organizations together. I think that was a hugely important event in the late 1970s and early 1980s.

Weaver: Can you tell us who and where, or details of how that came about?

Warren: I assume everybody remembers the Wendy Savage events in 1985, when she was accused of endangering women.[84] I think she got a lot of support from the voluntary organizations and from the mothers in their care. And I think that was the beginning of those groups coming together, and working with health professionals and that has gone on since that time. Certainly, I was lucky enough to learn what I thought was a lot about breastfeeding, we heard about your research and took that forward to mothers at grassroots. Obviously, we were not knowledgeable in the way that you were, but working with women at the grassroots and having the pleasure of saying: 'Yes, this does help women', and seeing the satisfaction and joy that breastfeeding brought them, I think, made us all much more committed as time went on, and many of us have continued working with breastfeeding for a very long time. That was a hugely important time. I don't know if anybody else agrees with that, but I think it started a movement where mothers, midwives, and voluntary organizations started to work together and put women at the centre of what was going on.

Mrs Phyll Buchanan: I want to make a small point. I am now speaking from the Breastfeeding Network, but partly it is recalling experiences from when I was a junior midwife at the Simpson in 1978 and I think it was the height of medical intervention. Something that really struck me as a young midwife was the women coming into the labour wards for their routine shavings and enemas: some women would come in and look at you straight in the face, and you knew that they were from the National Childbirth Trust (NCT). More than that, their case notes actually had 'NCT' in red letters on the front. As a student, I thought there must be something in this, because they would sometimes challenge you.

---

[84] See Savage (1986; 2007).

Weaver: And how did that come about so early?

Palmer: I am not an expert on the NCT, there are many in this room, for the record, I gave birth in 1970 and 1972 and had no contact with the NCT. But in 1972 I found a leaflet for the newly formed NCT breastfeeding promotion group in an NHS mother and baby clinic. I joined because I thought what a wonderful idea it was for women to help each other. I could not have afforded to pay for any breastfeeding counselling training but I got good free training from the NCT. I was given Mavis Gunther's *Infant Feeding*, which changed my life.[85]

At that time there was some hostility towards health professionals by some NCT women, and some would say vice versa. My local health visitor used me to give breastfeeding classes and support to local women.

Weaver: We are going to stop for tea in a few minutes. I wanted to get to the bottom of this: WHO and the Baby Friendly Initiative saw the interest in birth spacing as separate from the interest in feeding.[86] When did WHO properly connect these together?

Akre: Things were done a bit backwards, because I don't think WHO as an organization understood the implications of everything that we have been talking about for the last two hours. In fact, what precipitated the whole push towards the *International Code of Marketing of Breast-milk Substitutes* goes back to the 1974 and 1978 Health Assembly resolutions and the 1979 meeting, which made a number of recommendations, including that there should be an international code.[87] This seemed to focus mainly on developing countries because of the deleterious impact of marketing and promotion of breast-milk substitutes in these environments, and therefore in 1981 the WHO's international code was adopted, following its drafting jointly with UNICEF and, of course, with the

---

[85] Gunther (1970).

[86] DoH/UNICEF UK Baby Friendly Initiative (1993).

[87] Mr James Akre wrote: 'In October 1979 WHO and UNICEF held their landmark joint meeting on infant and young child feeding in Geneva, attended by some 150 representatives of governments, nongovernmental organizations, professional associations, scientists and manufacturers of infant foods. Discussions centered on five themes: encouragement and support of breastfeeding; promotion and support of appropriate and timely complementary feeding; strengthening of education, training and information on infant and young child feeding; promotion of the health and social status of women in this connection; and appropriate marketing and distribution of breast-milk substitutes. Participants in the October 1979 meeting included Dr Elisabet Helsing, Professor Dick Jelliffe and Professor Pat Jelliffe. Baby Milk Action was a founding member of IBFAN, several of whose members also participated in the WHO/UNICEF meeting in October 1979.' Note on draft transcript, 7 October 2008.

participation of many organizations, including the activist groups, with some of the very representatives present here today.[88] After focusing on the marketing and promotion of breast-milk substitutes, it was only in 1989 with the publication of a joint statement on breastfeeding and maternity services that the role of maternity services was directly considered, with the launching in 1991 of the Baby-friendly Hospital Initiative.[89] Here we are in 2007, with last year's release of the new growth reference standard.[90] So, in a sense, all of it was done backwards, but the impetus, historically, came from what was happening in developing countries before being broadened to include all children, everywhere. Now we are talking about what's right for our species, and what's physiologically appropriate feeding behaviour. So, I think it is like looking through a telescope through the wrong end.

Weaver: Felicity, I don't know when you joined WHO, but what are your recollections of this period?

Savage: I joined WHO in 1993 but I had been doing consultancies for WHO and UNICEF for some years before that. LAM was a very strong influence on people's interest in breastfeeding in the 1980s, and, for a time, promotion of breastfeeding was emphasized in family planning programmes. Breastfeeding tends to have piggy-backed on other programmes. In the 1990s it became diarrhoeal disease control, when research showed that breastfeeding was the one provable way of preventing diarrhoea in children, particularly if they breastfed exclusively. Interest in breastfeeding was developing after the adoption of the *International Code of Marketing of Breast-milk Substitutes* in 1981, but then there was a lapse and there was little progress for several years, apart from the activity of groups who were promoting the implementation of the code. Then in 1986 UNICEF organized a meeting to discuss why so little was happening to promote breastfeeding. This was part of UNICEF's GOBI movement, which addressed **G**rowth monitoring, **O**ral rehydration, **B**reastfeeding and **I**mmunization.[91] The immunization and oral rehydration aspects were very successful but nothing was happening on breastfeeding, probably because

---

[88] WHO (1981b). Freely available at www.ibfan.org/site2005/Pages/article.php?art_id=52&iui=1 (visited 22 January 2009).

[89] See www.who.int/nutrition/topics/bfhi/en/index.html (visited 29 January 2009). See also Woolridge (1994); Broadfoot *et al.* (2005) and note 47.

[90] See www.who.int/childgrowth/standards/en (visited 13 October 2008).

[91] UNICEF introduced the GOBI strategy of four child health interventions in 1992. Birth spacing/family planning (F), food supplementation (F) and the promotion of female literacy (F) were added subsequently (GOBI-FFF). See Claeson and Waldman (2000).

it wasn't so easy to package. The UNICEF executive director, Jim Grant, asked a group of experts to suggest what could be done about breastfeeding. At about this time Michael Woolridge was researching the oral dynamics of milk transfer and we were beginning to understand how to help mothers to breastfeed. With the help of workers like Chloe Fisher, we were beginning to realize that many mothers need help to breastfeed effectively, and to understand how to help them. It took some time for this understanding to become more widespread. However, in 1989 a joint WHO/UNICEF statement, *Protecting, Promoting and Supporting Breastfeeding: The special role of maternity services,* was produced, which drew attention to the importance of healthcare practices, and gave us the *Ten Steps to Successful Breastfeeding,* which became the foundation of the Baby-friendly Hospital Initiative.[92] Subsequently, there was a series of meetings on all the different aspects of breastfeeding: one in Copenhagen on lactation management training organized by Elisabet Helsing, and others on mother support, women's employment, hospital practices, and the code. The conclusions of these meetings were presented at another meeting in WHO, Geneva on breastfeeding in the 1990s. This led to the Innocenti Declaration in 1991, at a meeting of policy makers in Florence, which was intended to make a recommendation for the Convention on the Rights of the Child in the same year.[93] The Innocenti Declaration led to the concept and implementation of the Baby-friendly Hospital Initiative.

Weaver: So, these were different sections in WHO that were coming together now and again with these meetings that were sponsored by WHO?

Savage: Yes, there was UNICEF; the nutrition division in WHO, which took a very leading role in the Baby Friendly Hospital Initiative; and the Diarrhoeal Disease Control Programme, which was also promoting breastfeeding for the prevention of diarrhoeal disease. They were separate divisions but contributing to the same initiative.

---

[92] WHO/UNICEF (1989). The ten steps are listed at www.unicef.org/newsline/tenstps.htm (visited 14 August 2008).

[93] The Innocenti Declaration was produced and adopted at the WHO/UNICEF policymakers' meeting, *Breastfeeding in the 1990s: A Global Initiative,* co-sponsored by the US Agency for International Development and the Swedish International Development Authority, at the Spedale degli Innocenti, Florence, Italy, 30 July – 1 August 1990. Freely available online at www.unicef.org/programme/breastfeeding/innocenti.htm (visited 22 January 2009). The infant formula and follow-on formula regulations came into force in the UK on 1 March 1995 to implement Commission Directive 91/321/EEC; see www.opsi.gov.uk/si/si1995/Uksi_19950077_en_1.htm (visited 22 January 2009).

Weaver: This was GOBI?

Savage: That was a UNICEF initiative.

Weaver: I see, and was that when the public health significance of breastfeeding with all its positive effects came together?

Savage: Yes, throughout the 1980s, these public health aspects began to come together and the activity started with the preparatory meeting that led to the Innocenti Declaration and the Convention on the Rights of the Child.

Rundall: I am sorry if my comment gave a misleading impression about this funding.[94] But, leaving aside the funding of the Gambia research, I do know that there has certainly been some funding from the infant feeding industry going into the MRC Dunn Nutrition Laboratory, Cambridge. I don't want to be disrespectful about people's intentions when they do research. It's obvious that all researchers are trying to find solutions and trying to find the correct situation impartially. And, the later work carried out by the Dunn was extremely valuable.[95] So it has been very interesting for me to hear all this, because, as I said, in the late 1970s–1980 we came in and did pick up on what WHO and the World Health Assembly were saying.

What was absolutely crucial for us was the evidence that babies were dying and that appalling practices were being carried out by the baby food industry. We were monitoring this, and we mustn't forget that. IBFAN was formed in 1980 and action groups running the Nestlé boycott triggered much of this concern to look at what was happening with breastfeeding and to look at what was called 'commerciogenic malnutrition' and actively do something about it. I think that if the consumer groups had not exerted pressure like that, the code would not have happened. It was essential to do something to try to stop the companies from doing positive harm. I can remember in 1980 wondering why health workers in developing countries didn't do something, didn't recognize what the problem was. I met a midwife at the first IBFAN meeting. She said: 'Babies die and we don't know why.' She said she was getting the milk companies in to do the training of the mothers, and was so rushed off her feet she didn't realise the harm. She just got them in to help. It was only when she got an IBFAN questionnaire she realized that this was the cause of the problem. The wrong

---

[94] See page 16.

[95] Mrs Patti Rundall wrote: 'My point is that inappropriate funding can have a damaging impact and can silence those who should speak out.' Note on draft transcript, 3 September 2007.

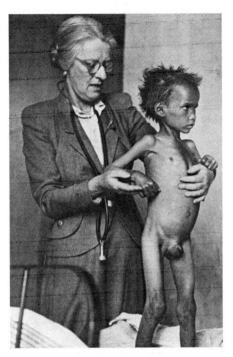

Figure 8: Dr Cicely Williams in India, 1950, with severely malnourished child.

people were giving the advice in the healthcare system. Elisabet is quite right about that; the healthcare systems were being invaded, even after the WHO code came in the companies took the code and pretended that they were behind it, which, of course, they were not. But they went all over the world promoting their versions of the code. Some of these companies had about 11 versions, confusing people and trying to get in as partners to help healthcare systems manage breastfeeding.

Weaver: And Cicely Williams? Nobody has mentioned her. We always read about her work being very much earlier, making these points.

Short: I am glad Cicely has been mentioned because I think she played an enormous role.[96] She was working in West Africa and brought to public attention that lovely West African word 'kwashiorkor', which means 'the evil eye of the child in the womb, upon the child already born'. What a prophetic statement. It wasn't invented by her, it was an indigenous term throughout Nigeria and much of the rest of West Africa; it was saying that if you have too short a birth interval, the new pregnancy switches off the milk supply to the older child, who will die

---

[96] See Williams (1933; 1935); Dally (1968).

of malnutrition. I will never forget going for the first time to Port au Prince, in Haiti, to the antenatal ward and looking at a row of about 20 mothers with their children. All the mothers were pregnant, coming for an antenatal examination, and there wasn't a single sound from any of their children. The obstetrician who was running the clinic said to me: 'You see those children? They will all be dead within six months. They have all got kwashiorkor.' I could see with my own eyes the evil eye of the child in the womb upon the child already born and how a short birth interval was having a disastrous effect. This was known in the developing world long before we discovered it. [97]

Weaver: Well, that's a sombre note on which to end the first half of this meeting.

Akre: To get in under the wire, because we are moving into another area, I would like to confirm what Patti Rundall has said. The international code would never have gone anywhere, it would never have got off the ground, if it hadn't been for the activist groups. So, we went from the particular to the collective summary of knowledge and awareness in international public health policy terms; from the international code in 1981 to the adoption of the *Global Strategy for Infant and Young Child Feeding* in May 2002. [98] And even if it's not going to win any literature prizes, I think that the global strategy pulls together all the disparate bits that we have talked about, and is the result of all the research activities that we have also discussed. In terms of public health policy, it was a combination of these events that was driving what WHO as an international organization was able to produce. So, things started with the particular, but ended with a much broader approach, the global strategy, which is now being implemented in over 160 countries.

Weaver: We are going to move on now in the second half to think, talk, or hear more about what happened in the UK in maternity units, neonatology units and what the neonatologists were doing. I am going to ask Dr Anthony Williams to start us off.

Dr Anthony Williams: I am going to give a slightly personal perspective as a way of introducing the area. I qualified as a doctor in 1975, so as a medical student and a young junior doctor in paediatric wards, the kind of practices we have heard about earlier today were very familiar to me, and I well remember the

---

[97] See also Reynolds and Tansey (eds) (2001b): 38.

[98] The global strategy was formally published in 2003, see WHO (2003).

babies being congregated in nurseries for several hours a day, rather than with their mothers. It's clear when you look at the texts of the 1970s and the early 1980s even, that many paediatricians were very supportive at least of the use of breast-milk in the neonatal units. I am thinking about the *Medical Care of Newborn Babies*, the Hammersmith textbook, which was perhaps the first big British textbook of neonatology.[99] I remember as a senior house officer in the 1970s in Leicester, David Davies, who unfortunately isn't able to be here today, being very pro the use of breast-milk for the babies and opening a breast-milk bank in Leicester. Of course, this was the era of setting up breast-milk banks in a sense, and there are names like Harold Gamsu, David Harvey, Brian Wharton with Sue Balmer in Birmingham and David Baum, to whom we shall come back later.[100]

As a registrar in Liverpool I hardly saw any breastfeeding in the late 1970s, and that reminds me of something quite important. I did my neonatal training in a very poor area on the edge of Liverpool and perhaps something that we haven't explicitly said is that the way a mother feeds her baby is probably the strongest measure of social and educational inequality that we have. Beth Alder referred to the resurgence being in social class I mothers and there is still that very wide divide. One of the important things that came out of the quinquennial *Infant Feeding Survey* statistics, at least in recent years, is that the gap has narrowed a bit.[101] It is the women in the lower social classes who have shown some resurgence in recent years. Also there's been resurgence outside England: in Scotland, to which Jenny Warren could attest, and in Northern Ireland and in Wales.

To come back to my career, I went from Liverpool to Oxford, and there I was extremely privileged to work with David Baum for about the next seven or eight years. Of course, there I also met Chloe Fisher. I must say that virtually anything I know about breastfeeding, I have learnt from midwives, most of whom are in this room. In my bag today I have still got my copy of *Successful Breastfeeding* [Figure 9], which I think Chloe, Ellena Salariya and other midwives here were instrumental in designing. As a result of that contact, I feel I know a little bit more about the practical aspects of breastfeeding than I otherwise would as a doctor.

---

[99] Davies *et al.* (1972).

[100] Sloper and Baum (1974); Baum (1979).

[101] See Table 1, page 9; Bolling *et al.* (2007); www.babyfriendly.org.uk/page.asp?page=21 (visited 17 June 2008).

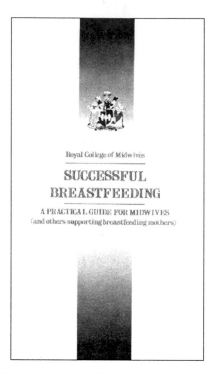

Figure 9: The Royal College of Midwives' practical guide, 1988.

I was disappointed only quite recently to be teaching a group of senior specialist registrars, one of whom was about to become a consultant in neonatal medicine, about the mechanics of breastfeeding. He told me that this was the first teaching he had ever had on breastfeeding in his entire training, so we still have a considerable training gap in medical practice, and particularly with neonatologists. In neonatology we have lost the sense of the general paediatrician. David Baum was an example of somebody who was first and foremost a general paediatrician and secondly a neonatologist, so he was able to see vividly the wider importance of breastfeeding. There are other neonataologists that I could mention again in that context. We have got Forrester Cockburn and Edmund Hey here. The problem with many current neonatologists, I think, speaking as one, is that they are much more focused on the care of the sick newborn. They go from an intensive care unit to the normal newborn baby in hospital. This produces a feeling that a baby has 'requirements', which must be met on 'day one' and 'day two' and so on. So we are almost back to the prescriptive: 'one minute on the first day', 'two minutes on the second day' and so on. People want to stick things in the baby and measure numbers to make sure the baby has got enough milk to prevent him or her falling apart within the first week of life. So there is still, I think, a gap to be bridged where neonatologists are concerned in terms of appreciating the difference between the normal newborn baby and the baby in a neonatal unit. Perhaps I shouldn't speak for them, but I think that can apply to some neonatal nurses as well.

To go back to the 1980s for a minute, I was privileged to work with people also like Mike Woolridge on the opposite side of the room here, and to learn about the science of breast-milk transfer.[102] We really began to understand a number of things about that, and in many respects I think this has been the least well-studied aspect of breastfeeding – how milk actually gets from the mother into the baby. A lot of light was shed on that process in the 1980s, much of it, I have to say, underpinning what Mavis Gunther had been saying very much earlier in her book.[103] But we have, if you like, a fuller scientific validation now. It was also a time at which there was a lot of interest in learning about breastfeeding, and Mike Woolridge, Chloe Fisher and I remember that we were probably spending a considerable amount of time, often at weekends, going to 'breastfeeding roadshows' and study days in postgraduate centres up and down the country, which were usually crowded out with midwives eager to learn more about breastfeeding. The later publication of *Successful Breastfeeding* was an indication of that thirst, if you like, for the knowledge amongst the midwifery community.

The final thing I would like to discuss, because it hasn't been mentioned in any depth so far, is the Baby Friendly Initiative in the UK.[104] We went through a couple of national initiatives, with the Department of Health, in the early 1990s. There was the Joint Breastfeeding Initiative, and then the National Breastfeeding Working Group, and that gave rise to the National Infant Feeding Coordinators later.[105] About 1992/3 the Baby Friendly Initiative began in the UK, and, again, it was David Baum together with Robert Smith at UNICEF

---

[102] See Woolridge (1986).

[103] Gunther (1970). See page 40.

[104] See note 47.

[105] The Minister of Health, Edwina Currie MP, challenged health professionals and voluntary organizations, in 1987, to work together to promote and support breastfeeding, resulting in the Joint Breastfeeding Initiative in England in 1987 and in Scotland in 1990. In England, the National Breastfeeding Working Group was established by the Department of Health in 1992 and produced guidance for the NHS in 1995 [National Breastfeeding Working Group (1995); Campbell and Jones (1994)]. For details of subsequent development in Scotland, Wales and Northern Ireland see www.scotland.gov.uk/Publications/2006/04/03092034/8 (visited 19 February 2009); DoH, Scottish Office (1996); The National Assembly for Wales (2001); DHSS (2004).

who were the driving forces in getting that initiative going in the UK. Mike Woolridge may be able to speak about this again as the first programme director of the Baby Friendly Initiative in the UK. Now this initiative did many things for breastfeeding, I think. One of the most important was that it began the 'big tent' for breastfeeding, where everybody could join in, and it dealt to some extent with the divisions that there might have been between the healthcare professionals, the mothers and everybody else. It almost provided, if you like, a brand for breastfeeding, which was necessary in some respects in a partly commercialized world. There's no doubt from the international work that has been done that the Baby-friendly Hospital Initiative is an extremely successful way of increasing the proportion of mothers breastfeeding and reducing preventable disease in the community. For example, the Belarus study was the strongest evidence of that from a large-cluster randomized trial.[106]

I also think that in the UK we have some very good data that show how effective the UNICEF Baby Friendly Initiative has been here. One of the great contributors to that, I think, has been the precision and the accuracy of the data that's been collected in Scotland. It was Forrester Cockburn who published the paper on the use of Guthrie cards to document whether women are breastfeeding at the end of the first week.[107] We still don't have that kind of population data in the other countries and it's sorely needed. The Baby Friendly Initiative also has been an unappreciated vehicle for midwifery training if you look at what the initiative has done in its 10 or 12 years. I think I heard it's trained thousands of midwives and also junior doctors in hospitals that have become 'baby friendly'. So it's undertaken a huge task and the fact that we now have something like 60 or more Baby Friendly hospitals in the UK is evidence of that. I remember when it started off in the 1990s people were asking why we were bothering with the Baby Friendly Initiative in the UK. The testimony is that we have over 60 hospitals, and many more working towards it, with certificates of commitment. I think

---

[106] Kramer *et al.* (2001).

[107] Professor Laurence Weaver wrote: 'Robert Guthrie was the inventor of a method for neonatal screening for phenylketonuria'. Note on draft transcript, 20 October 2008. Professor Forrester Cockburn wrote: 'Guthrie cards are used in Britain to screen all babies for inherited metabolic disease and hypothyroidism. District midwives take blood from the heels of every baby seven days after birth and test it on the specially absorbent card. They also routinely record on the card the feeding method used on the day the infant is seen, the date of birth and address (including postcode) and the hospital of birth; only one method of feeding, bottle or breast, is recorded as there is no scope for recording mixed feeding.' Ferguson *et al.* (1994): 824. See also Tappin *et al.* (1991; 1993); Guthrie (1996).

that's all I would like to say now and I will open this up for discussion. There are things I haven't mentioned, like the successive Committee on Medical Aspects of Food and Nutrition Policy (COMA) reports, the grey books and the people who were involved in producing those, but perhaps we can pick those up later.[108]

Weaver: You mentioned a number of topics that I think we would like to pursue. I want to get back as early as possible historically, to the early 1970s. You and I both qualified at about the same time and you said how our seniors were not really interested in breastfeeding, except for one or two who are here, so maybe we will put the spotlight on Forrester Cockburn.

Professor Forrester Cockburn: I was also in the Simpson Memorial Maternity Pavilion, Edinburgh, but I had left by the time most of the work that Roger Short and the others were talking about.[109] One of the things that I remember from the 1960s was, at that time, particularly after the withdrawal of National Dried Milk, individual milk companies had contracts for the milk kitchens in each of the major maternity units in this country.[110] Each firm jealously guarded and argued the need for its particular brand of milk to be in that hospital and there were financial and other inducements, which had a major adverse effect on breastfeeding to which paediatricians paid insufficient attention.[111] One has to remember that there were virtually no paediatricians in the late 1950s and early 1960s dealing full-time with the newborn.[112] There was the occasional consultant visit from the nearby children's hospital, with a few exceptions like Bristol and Birmingham. The whole attitude was not influenced by neonatal paediatricians because there weren't any so-called neonatal paediatricians before about 1968, when paediatricians with knowledge of the physiology and biochemistry of the newborn human infant began to appear for the first time.

I got involved partly because I was interested in inherited metabolic disease and knew something about physiology and biochemistry. My interest in neonatal nutrition started with phenylketonuria, because after 1957, when the treatment of phenylketonuria was introduced, we had to produce a good infant milk with a low protein, low phenylalanine and reasonable tyrosine levels. None of the

---

[108] DHSS (1977; 1980); DoH (1994).

[109] See pages 29–32.

[110] See Glossary, page 128. See also Oppé *et al.* (1974); Baum and Harker (1975); Arneil *et al.* (1975).

[111] See Church and Tansey (2007): 370–1.

[112] See Walker-Smith (1997).

milks available at that time, which were largely high-protein, caseine-based, were of much use. I was in the US working on the type of diet that might best be suited to the infant with phenylketonuria. We showed that whey protein was perhaps a better material on which to base infant formulae for children with metabolic diseases generally, but in particular phenylketonuria. When I came back to Edinburgh, I think it was Ron Hendey who got hold of my data and instead of feeding whey protein to pigs, they decided to feed it to human beings and stop using whole or caseine-based milks.[113]

When I came back to Edinburgh as a Wellcome senior research fellow from Oxford, a major problem of the time was neonatal convulsions. Every winter in the Simpson we had several hundred babies convulsing merrily, half of them through hypoxia induced by various obstetric complications and the other half due to hypocalcaemia and/or hypomagnesaemia, and the next biochemical exercise was to work out what was happening. We found that the women in Edinburgh at that time were vitamin D-deficient during the later winter/early spring, and I think they still are today, and that this was the reason for the seasonal prevalence of convulsions in the newborn, and that the high-phosphate milks were the trigger to the convulsions.[114] So I spent the rest of my life telling milk companies that their products were biochemical rubbish as far as the human infant was concerned. My latest research involved looking at the lipids in the milk and showing that the composition of the brain of the human infant that has been fed on cow milk formulae is completely different from that of breastfed infants.[115] There is a real need for formula milks for some infants and for safe breast-milk substitutes, so my role has been that of being devil's advocate.

One little thing about the WHO and its code was that for a while we had what was called the Code Monitoring Committee in the UK and the chairman was Dame Alison Munro, who was quite formidable.[116] As a point of historical

---

[113] See Janas *et al.* (1985).

[114] Cockburn *et al.* (1973).

[115] See Farquharson *et al.* (1992; 1995).

[116] The *International Code of Practice* [WHO (1981b)] was introduced in the UK in 1983 and was supported by a Code Monitoring Committee on infant formulae consisting of eight members nominated by the Government, four nominated by the Food Manufacturers Federation and Government-nominated chairman Dame Alison Munro (1985–89). The code bans advertising to the general public except under the control of the healthcare system and controls advertising to health professionals themselves. The committee considers complaints against the international code.

interest, her brother was Ian Donald, who introduced ultrasound to medicine.[117] She tried hard to keep the cartload of monkeys called the Food Manufacturers Federation under control. But only four of the milk firms were involved and eventually the whole thing fizzled out. I was on the committee at that time and we eventually agreed to accept the whole of the WHO code.[118] These are just a few of my thoughts, but Edmund Hey was involved in another aspect of milk, infant hypernatraemia, but he says: 'No, it wasn't hypernatraemia.' Perhaps he could carry on from here with that aspect of things that frightened women about artificially feeding their babies.

Weaver: Yes, Edmund, please. I was your senior house officer in the late 1970s and I remember being taught nothing about infant feeding at all.

Hey: No, I didn't teach you anything about infant feeding. The control of feeding was in the hands of the nursing staff and even in the premature babies they would dictate who was fed, how and when, and they knew how to do it. It was not a medical issue at all. It was kept from the medical staff. The nursing staff would decide when to start, when to stop and how much to give. I really think that we should never have entered the field, that is my view. I spent my time encouraging the nurses that this was an area where they really did know better and if they could only think of scientific reasons rather than just say: 'Well, because I know it's true', they would actually earn the respect of the medical staff, the confidence of the women and keep this as something that women can teach women better. What's nursing about? It's a strange word, isn't it.[119] And a skill that midwives should have retained all along. We as neonatologists should never have entered into it.

I wasn't a neonatologist; I tried to be a paediatrician. Yes, I do recall being in Newcastle at the stage when milks contained too much phosphate and also

---

[117] See Tansey and Christie (eds) (2000); Willocks and Barr (2004).

[118] Mrs Patti Rundall wrote: 'Professor Cockburn refers to the monitoring committee fizzling out and then going straight to the whole of the WHO code. Sadly this wasn't the case. The UK has never implemented the whole code and has allowed advertising to persist to this day. An NCT/UNICEF survey carried out in 2005 showed the impact of this marketing and found more than one-third of mothers thought that the advertising conveyed the message that formula was "as good" or "better than" breast-milk.' Letter to Dr Daphne Christie, 3 September 2007. See NCT/UNICEF (2005), which includes details of the results of the 1000 telephone interviews conducted 16–22 August 2005.

[119] Dr Edmund Hey wrote: 'When someone spoke 200 years ago about a baby being "nursed" they were saying it was being fed, or suckled. It is sad to think that, although nurses have now acquired many new and invaluable skills, they seem to be at risk of losing the oldest one of all.' Note on draft transcript, 10 September 2007.

contained too much sodium, so that if the baby got the squitters, you ended up with hypernatraemia.[120] The early formula milks were pretty alarming when the baby's physiology was under stress. Even now, of course, people are worried about breastfeeding, the fact that if the intake isn't very good and the weight drops away, maybe the baby should be weighed every day. I am not sure what Dr Anthony Williams thinks about weighing at regular intervals, but there are 1 or 2 per cent of breastfed babies crashing into hospital with quite serious weight loss now, who are hypernatraemic and if you read some of the papers on the subject, they imply that it's because there's too much sodium in the milk that the mother is giving. It's all upside down. The problem is that the baby has not had enough water, not that it has had too much salt. It's the ratio that you are looking at. When you say: 'Oh dear, this baby has got high sodium.' No, he hasn't, he hasn't got enough water to dilute the sodium. I will end at that point. I really do think that this is an area that should be de-medicalized, and I am glad to see a whole host of midwives here today.

Weaver: Mike Woolridge, it has been suggested that you would tell us more about Baby Friendly issues.

Woolridge: I could do, but I simply wanted to say that I actually arrived in this field as an interloper, because I have no medical allegiance, I am not medically qualified, I am not a paediatrician or an obstetrician; I am a zoologist, somebody who has never been involved in veterinary practice or dairy science. It occurred to me when I arrived that paediatricians have a responsibility and an interest in the newborn, so they study the newborn in isolation. Obstetricians, to a certain extent, seem to study the mother and her makeup in isolation. The zoologist looks at the interaction between the two animals as perfectly natural, so I found it very easy to look at the interaction between mothers and babies. I suppose I was gratified scientifically to see that the research going on in Edinburgh and Cambridge was at least looking at the process of the interaction between mother and baby, rather than looking at milk output of dairy animals. That is not to disparage that at all, but animal research was something that I was never familiar with or comfortable with.

Weaver: So how did you take up the reins of the Baby Friendly Initiative?

Woolridge: Well, I don't know how, but with horror, because my initial reaction was that this was a very rigid, prescriptive scheme that would be imposed on

---

[120] Anand *et al.* (2002); Morton (1989); Oddie *et al.* (2001); Laing and Wong (2002); Richmond (2003); Iyer *et al.* (2007); Crossland *et al.* (2008).

women and I thought it would be received with a degree of unrest. However, the more I looked into it and the more I found that it was delivered in a sympathetic, more flexible way, the more I came to appreciate its potential benefits. I suppose in the early days of the Baby Friendly Initiative in this country it was developed and implemented in a very flexible manner. I think, looking at the national data, I would currently attribute the most recent change from 2000 to 2005 to the impact of national policy changes through the Baby Friendly Initiative, not governmentally introduced, but through this sort of overall cultural impact of the UK Baby Friendly Initiative. Looking back to 1975–80, I don't think it was professionally induced change, I think it was a cultural revolution that was taking place. I know Elisabet will probably acknowledge that in Europe what is called a Green Wave led to a cultural shift in the population, and although a lot of people would like to claim credit for it, I think it is a largely independent cultural change amongst women, probably supported and encouraged by lay support groups.[121]

Howie: I'm from Dundee. We have been talking about neonatal paediatricians but not much about obstetricians, of which I am one. Of course, the obstetricians do have quite an important influence on women in the antenatal and immediate postnatal period. When I went to Dundee I took my interest in breastfeeding from Edinburgh but was told repeatedly by my colleagues that I should not pursue it because I was making their patients feel guilty. This has not been mentioned very much, but I was told that mothers who were inclined initially to choose to bottle-feed should not be leant upon or persuaded because if they continued to bottle-feed and make that their choice, they would feel guilty. Indeed, that was a major stimulus for undertaking the infant feeding and health study, which may be appropriate to talk about later on.[122] Many of my colleagues said: 'And in any case, it doesn't make the slightest difference at the end of the day whether the mother bottle-feeds or breastfeeds.' When I went to Edinburgh in the late 1980s, I would have said that was the predominant attitude amongst obstetricians, and also amongst quite a lot of midwives. Many other midwives took an exact opposite feeling and were very enthusiastic about breastfeeding, but I think midwives, if they are honest, would say that they were divided. But this 'don't make the mothers feel guilty' was a very powerful motive.

---

[121] See Rosenberg (1989).

[122] See Howie *et al.* (1990) and pages 74–5.

Salariya: I concur with Peter Howie's thoughts about people being against breastfeeding. As a student midwife in Glasgow in the 1950s, and later in Dundee as a staff midwife, one had to be on one's guard about mentioning breastfeeding, as bottle-feeding mothers would feel guilty. Supplementary and complementary bottle-feeds of formula milk were given to the breastfed infants secretly by midwives and nursing staff. When my first baby was born in 1954 I insisted that he remain in the room with me at all times. I was not popular and was considered somewhat of a rebel, but I simply could not trust the staff that he would not receive formula milk. I breastfed the baby when he needed to be fed and had no problems.

Later, as a community midwife, I advised mothers at home to breastfeed their babies as soon after delivery as was practical. I personally supervised the initial latching-on process and had no problems. The infants passed meconium early and we never admitted a breastfed infant to hospital because of 'jaundice' or excessive weight loss or dehydration.

During the 1960s I was appointed sister in the labour suite at Dundee Royal Infirmary. This was when intra partum continuous monitoring was in its infancy using Hewlett-Packard machines. Obstetricians and midwives were fascinated with the new technology and some of the midwives even began to have screwdrivers in the top pockets of their uniforms, to adjust the temperamental apparatus when required.

I helped a mother to deliver her baby – she indicated that she was keen to give breastfeeding a try and when I enquired when this could be initiated I was told 'we certainly do not have the time to be bothered with that in the labour suite'. I was then made aware of the 'regime'. There was the one minute at each side performance six to eight hours post-delivery – nothing had changed!

I indicated that I was interested in carrying out some research and requested to be appointed to a postnatal ward at the same hospital. It does seem unrealistic now that my argument that the lactation process and what was being carried out in practice did not make sense and my request was rejected by both medical and midwifery hierarchy.

After discussion with newly delivered mothers and ward midwives we began to initiate breastfeeding whenever the mothers arrived from the labour suite after delivery. A member of ward staff 'guarded' the ward entrance and mothers were 'screened off' to begin with. After a time the screens were not used and several bottle-feeding mothers in the Nightingale ward requested to change to breastfeeding. The ward midwives became very competitive about their abilities to assist with the initial latching-on process, although it was still being done in 'secret'.

One day a new consultant paediatrician, Dr John Cater, came to do a ward round after visiting the other two postnatal wards. As he was about to leave he enquired: 'Is this the breastfeeding ward?' I simply could not believe my ears and immediately thought: 'Oh – this is my man.' He later listened to my 'theory' and said: 'Prove it.' I received my greatest encouragement from John and I shall be forever grateful for his wise and learned counselling.

I was asked to speak at a 'medical' meeting later at Ninewells Hospital about breastfeeding and was in great awe. I asked my brother, a medic, what he had been taught as a student about the subject – he thought for a moment and replied: 'A baby requires two and a half ounces of milk per pound of body weight per day'. End of story.

I went on to carry out a study showing that the earlier a baby is put to the breast and the more frequently he is fed during the early days, the longer breastfeeding will continue to take place.[123]

Hey: The important thing to say is that she got that paper published in the *Lancet*.

Weaver: Why didn't that paper influence midwives elsewhere?

Hey: Because they don't read the *Lancet*, but it did have an impact on the medical profession, a really profound one. I want to know who encouraged you to go for the *Lancet*. It was a monumental step.

Salariya: It was suggested by John Cater that I offer it to the *Lancet* for publication. I received a 'nice' letter rejecting the study, saying that as I wasn't a medical practitioner they could not accept it. So John decided to be the third named author and that's how we got it into the *Lancet* in 1978. Again, I thank Dr Cater.

Weaver: Now, the midwives please. I want to know why the professionals were not taking up these ideas. Why this wasn't happening elsewhere? Or how did it start happening elsewhere?

Renfrew: I will start, but there are many others with lots of stories. I think there was a great division in midwifery, where you were aligned either with wanting

---

[123] Salariya *et al.* (1978).

to pick up ideas like this, or you were kind of stuck with what you had been taught. The sheer power, the dominance, of the timed feeds and the separation between mothers and babies was fiercely difficult to shift. I remember many, many occasions when I was working with my colleagues from the MRC – I had a joint appointment in the Simpson – I went round the postnatal wards, trying to say: 'Can't we stop the timing? Can we stop using the Rotersept spray, because that's actually not going to stop the sore nipples? Can't we just have mothers with babies?' And there was a sheer weight of dominance that was partly from the midwives who were responsible for the wards, but here my experience is different from Ed Hey's; the pressure was also from the paediatricians, who really wanted to see this kind of absolute medicalized policy in place. It wasn't just Ellena's work that people were ignoring. The demand feeding-paper by Illingworth and Stone that was published in 1952 had made no impact either.[124] We came later to review the papers for what became *Effective Care in Pregnancy and Childbirth* and then the Cochrane Collaboration pregnancy and childbirth reviews.[125] When we started reviewing this, it was amazing to find the Illingworth and Stone paper from 1952 and other papers that had been out there quite a long time that hadn't made it through into practice.

I actually think one of the reasons it didn't make a difference was that people didn't know how to do it. They actually didn't know about positioning [Figure 10] – I am going to hand this microphone to Chloe in a minute. They didn't know that you could put a baby to the breast so it didn't hurt.[126] I think a common experience for midwives was they gave the baby to the mother, the mother tried to put the baby to the breast and it hurt like heck, and they actually didn't know what to do about that. Therefore they needed the Rotersept, because their nipples were getting sore. Therefore you had to time the feeds so the nipples didn't get sore. It was all self-perpetuating. And you had to be really lucky to work with a practitioner like Ellena or Chloe, who somehow had figured this out for themselves. How did you do it?

Fisher: Very difficult to say. I qualified in 1956 and I was not going to be a midwife unless I could be a midwife outside of hospitals. What I saw happening to mothers and babies in my part two training had me cycling home crying.

---

[124] Illingworth *et al.* (1952).

[125] Chalmers *et al.* (eds) (1989). For details of the Cochrane Collaboration, see www.cochrane.org/evidenceaid/pregnancyandchildbirth/ (visited 7 August 2008); see also Reynolds and Tansey (eds) (2005).

[126] See Figure 5, page 18.

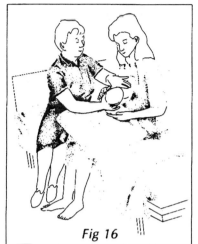
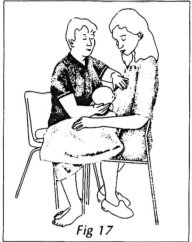

Having attached the baby correctly, the mother can then
be encouraged to relax her back and shoulders against
the supporting chair. A footstool may also be a useful
aid to relaxation.

Figure 10: Positioning the baby correctly. From the Royal College of Midwives'
practical guide, *Successful Breastfeeding*, 1988.

I thought: 'If I can't do something about this, then I am going to take up horticulture.' Anyway, I then did my experience training in the home and found it a totally different experience. When I first started among the women in Oxford who had delivered at home – that was 40 per cent of our population – 85 per cent of them were exclusively breastfeeding at two weeks, compared with institutional deliveries of 76 per cent. So, if you see, where I came from, where it was simply normal to breastfeed, this was in Oxford, the population I was working with, the dons and in the slums, everybody breastfed. As a midwife, if a woman had a problem I had the responsibility to sort it out. It never occurred to me that breastfeeding wasn't as important as giving birth.

Weaver: And how would you assume that responsibility?

Fisher: Intuition – no, I mean it wasn't official – but just because I was a midwife, and as a domiciliary midwife I was responsible for my mothers for 14 days after delivery, and if they intended to breastfeed and they had a problem, I had to try to figure out how to help them. That's when I first got on to the importance of correctly attaching babies to the breast. I began to think that this was incredibly important, and I absolutely couldn't understand why everybody didn't know about it.

Weaver: Did you work in an environment where there wasn't infant formula in the lying-in ward?

Fisher: I was working in women's homes. I always remained community-based. Just one little story, because I could go on for ever. When we started having official early discharges from the hospitals, which was happening in the 1960s, we were starting to have healthy women coming home for most of their care. I could take you to the house still where a mother was allowing her beautiful large baby to stay on the breast precisely ten minutes and then topping it up with formula as she had been advised by the hospital. She had gallons of milk in her breasts. It just reminded me how awful breastfeeding practice in hospital was, and I am afraid I have sat on the edge of it ever since.[127] I have always been community-based. I haven't done what anybody else has told me to do, but I have worked with the mothers and with the babies and done my absolute best to solve problems for them and then they go on to continue to breastfeed.

Helsing: Hospitals were never made for births and that certainly is the case in our country and maybe here too. I can see people nodding. And therefore the medical training is geared towards neither birth nor breastfeeding. In fact, it happened very slowly that births got into hospitals. It only began in my country, Norway – a typical middle-income European country at the time – around the middle of the nineteenth century, when the mothers-to-be found their way into the hospitals. But hospital routines are for sick people and women who give birth are not sick. In health workers' training, breastfeeding was simply not an issue. Health workers consequently were of the opinion that either mothers managed to breastfeed or they didn't, and if they didn't, it was just too bad, and that was the end of the story. I am sorry to say that health workers were not too helpful in the resurgence of breastfeeding, at least in Scandinavia. Mother-led resurgence of breastfeeding can be very successful and has been in Norway [see Figure 11].

---

[127] Miss Chloe Fisher wrote: 'This is an example from the tragically misguided era during which mothers were urged to look at clocks instead of at their babies. It has its origin early in the twentieth century and, sadly, continues to this day, where it is now known as "traditional". Artificially imposed restrictions on the duration and frequency of feeds, practices which had become firmly rooted in most maternity hospitals, must have played a major part in the rapid decline in the incidence of breastfeeding in the 1960s, which was when women were urged to give birth in hospital instead of at home.' Note on draft transcript, 4 September 2007. See Appendix 1; Woolridge and Ingram (2007).

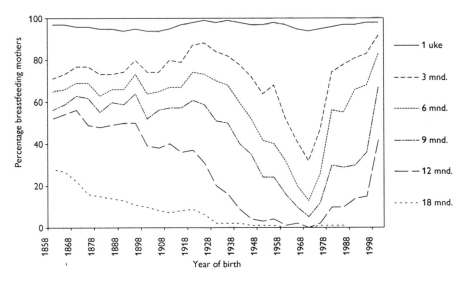

Figure 11: Breastfeeding uptake and duration in Norway, 1858 to 1998, in weeks (uke) and months (mnd).[128]

Savage: Before we move on too far, I would like to point out that Ellena Salariya's paper, the Illingworth paper and the publications by Chloe Fisher and others that have been mentioned may not have had an immediate impact on healthcare practices, but when they are all gathered together, these were very important background evidence on which the 'ten steps' were based.[129] If you say: 'Well, cut the doctors out, leave the midwives to it', the midwives are undoubtedly much better, but they need the support and leadership of doctors or by themselves they won't be able to make the necessary changes. So, doctors have to accept responsibility for not permitting the necessary changes to be introduced into policy and practice.

Professor Fiona Dykes: I'm from the University of Central Lancashire and also a midwife. I want to pick up on the notion of the power of the institution. I remember when I first trained as a midwife in the 1980s in Chatham, Kent,

---

[128] Data from 9150 women delivering in the major hospitals in Oslo, Bergen and Trondheim between 1858 and 1988 from mothers' responses to routine questions asked about their *previous* child [Rosenberg (1991)], using data originally published in Liestøl *et al.* (1988). Information updated for 1988–1998 from accessible data based on a representative selection of children in a number of provinces with some adjustments to take account of a 1998 nationwide study by the Norwegian Nutrition Council. See Lande (2003). Details of this study will be deposited along with other records of this meeting in archives and manuscripts, Wellcome Library, London, in GC/253.

[129] Illingworth *et al.* (1952); Salariya *et al.* (1978); Fisher (1985); Vallena and Savage (1998).

walking on to a Victorian-style, Florence Nightingale ward, where the women were lined up on either side of the ward and the whole emphasis was on orderliness and along the middle of the ward there were trolleys of milk and the noisy or disorderly babies were in a nursery.[130] The whole emphasis was on timing and control. There was a real fear of any sort of chaos, anything that disrupted orderliness, and I would suggest that this relates to very strong western values around the clock and timing. It's not surprising that the predominant icon in the UK is Big Ben. Even now, although we talk about demand feeding, there's still a sense of midwives going to women and saying: 'Oh, good, you are demand feeding. How often are you demand feeding? How long is the baby feeding for? But, good, you are feeding on demand.' Women are asking what demand feeding really means. So, you know, comparing what is understood in the UK to be demand feeding with the examples we have been given of the Aborigine communities, or the Kalahari Desert Wanderers, they are poles apart; and I feel it is important that we really understand the power of our culturally embedded desire for orderliness and timeliness.[131]

Weaver: Who was maintaining this culture in Chatham? The teacher–midwife? Why weren't the medical staff involved?

Dykes: It's broader than just the institution, it's deeply culturally based, but the hospital is based on a factory. If we look at the development of the hospital historically, it was very similar to the factory or even to the prison. Everybody could be seen, including the staff, including the people who were availing themselves of this service, and hospitals were run on sort of factory- or prison-based guidelines and that is deeply entrenched. I don't think you can single out any one disciplinary group, doctors, paediatricians or midwives. The factory principles were deeply culturally ingrained and everyone has been wrapped up in that particular institutional culture.[132]

Weaver: Well, there's a paediatrician here. Brian wants to say something.

Wharton: It's very interesting, very illuminating listening to what people have done and their own individual services, and we have all read a lot about what

---

[130] See note 38.

[131] See discussion on pages 22–3.

[132] See Baker (1956); Granshaw and Porter (1989); Gallivan (2000); www.nationalarchives.gov.uk/ERORecords/JA/4/1/Documents/Gallivanreportonmonitoringclinicalperformance (visited 8 July 2008).

they have done and learned from it. If you take an overall national view, there was a big change between 1975 and 1980, quite a substantial one and very little since 1980. So that would need some explanation. I agree that is perhaps not part of the Witness event that we are taking part in now, where we are all telling it as we saw it. I think we could get our optimistic blinkers on if we think all of these programmes which enthusiasts have introduced and have been very successful and which are having much national impact. Because I don't see that the figures support it. Nor do I understand why there was this great improvement between 1975 and 1980, a sense of euphoria, and then for some reason since 1980 the movements have been very, very small. As I say, statisticians think they are explained by other demographic changes.

Dr Alison Spiro: I am a health visitor and an anthropologist. I would just like to follow on from what Fiona was saying about the time constraints put on breastfeeding and where they all come from. I moved into anthropology because I felt I wasn't getting the answers through biomedicine as to why women weren't breastfeeding. I have done work with an Indian community in Harrow, the Gujarati community, and I have done work in India as well. Indian women I have spoken to say that there's no time for breastfeeding in this country. For them there are too many other things that impact on their lives, but in India there's time for breastfeeding. Here it's much more difficult. The other thing that I would like to say follows on from what Fiona said about the metaphors of production that we use. The terminology of supply and demand and a whole load of other examples show that the way we see breastfeeding is as a mechanistic transfer of milk from the mother to the baby. I think those of us who have been looking at breastfeeding all know that what goes on in the mother's social life is absolutely crucial to whether the baby actually gets the milk transferred.

In my work in anthropology, I found that breastfeeding pervades every single aspect of social life, whether it is gender relations, politics, rituals; the rituals about evil eye, the rituals about colostrum and lots of these things are very, very important. I think that we need to look at the whole context, not just the biomedical transfer of milk.

Ms Rosie Dodds: I'm from the National Childbirth Trust. I would like to pick up on what Professor Wharton was saying and Tony and Mike's references to the statistics on breastfeeding in this country. I think we have to turn the question on its head. There's so much evidence that we are now aware of about the major impact that breastfeeding has on each individual baby, but also on the mother from a public health perspective, and on the wider society, reducing inequalities in health. Many people now recognize the social class divide in this country, that women are more likely to breastfeed if they are older and if they have got more years of education, changes to that culture would do a lot to reduce health inequalities. Also, whether we are talking about breastfeeding in the UK, breastfeeding in England, or breastfeeding across the world, breastfeeding has been recognized as the most effective way to reduce child mortality. The deaths of 13 per cent of babies who die in the poorest countries, at least, could be prevented by breastfeeding, and further deaths could be prevented by adequate complementary feeding and continued breastfeeding.[133] So the question is not why breastfeeding increased in this country, but why breastfeeding rates are so low and why they are not increasing more. What are the influences, particularly following the point about the Baby Friendly Initiative, increasing breastfeeding rates in hospitals? And there's good evidence that this is the case.[134] We don't know yet the long-term impact in this country but evidence from Italy, Sweden and the Belarus studies show that the continuation rates are better there.[135] But will they be better in this country or is the social support and public support so poor that women really don't have a chance to carry on breastfeeding?

Michaelsen: A short comment: I am a paediatrician from Copenhagen working mainly with nutrition. Some years ago I wrote a book for WHO and UNICEF with Lawrence Weaver, Aileen Robertson and Francesco Branca on guidelines in infant feeding.[136] It was for the WHO European region, which also includes the former Soviet republics. We were exploring what the recommendations were in the Soviet Union. The recommendations on timing of breastfeeding were very strict. We have talked about rigid time limits here.[137] There the official recommendations were that you had to breastfeed every two hours for the first month, and then every three hours. We had a doctor from Lithuania helping us to explore the literature in Russian and she found a paper saying that perhaps you didn't have to be so rigid, that you could relax a bit from these time frames, and plus or minus 15 minutes would be all right.

---

[133] Jones *et al.* (2003): 67.

[134] Bartington *et al.* (2006).

[135] Cattaneo and Buzzetti (2001); Hofvander (2005); Kramer *et al.* (2001).

[136] Michaelsen *et al.* (eds) (2003).

[137] Pages 22–3, 62 and 64.

Weaver: Do you want to say anything about the International Society for Research in Human Milk and Lactation and how that came in from the side and brought together a new lot of people?

Michaelsen: That is the International Society of Research in Human Milk and Lactation, a very long name, also called ISRHML.[138] It was established in the 1980s as a research society and has always been a small one, with 200–300 members who meet every two years. The first two were in Costa Rica and California. There have been many meetings and for most of them there has been a book published which has had very useful background information on the research.[139] One of the last meetings was in Cambridge, arranged by Ann Prentice among others. Among those who have been involved in the society from the beginning are: Armond Goldman, Margit Hamosh, Stephanie Atkinson and Bo Lönnerdal. There was a recent meeting in Toronto and the next will be in Perth in February 2008. The society has mainly focused on physiological aspects, bioactive components in breast-milk and the effects on offspring and the mother. For the last one and a half years, we have given out bibliographies every three months, including titles and abstracts of all those publications on breastfeeding that appear on Medline.[140] They are freely available on our website. There is an impressive number of publications on breastfeeding, at least 50–60 relevant papers every month. We do not sort them according to quality, but classify them according to topic.

Weaver: Do you think the society has been influential or just a forum?

Michaelsen: It has been a small scientific society, so I think it's been influential on the science side, but it has not taken on the public-health aspect. They have tried to concentrate on the physiological or scientific aspects.

Hanson: A brief comment going back to the 1950s. When I started to collect my first breast-milk samples, it was rather difficult. I was regarded as a rather strange creature; why on earth would I be interested in human milk? Bovine milk would have been alright. Good nurses and midwives helped me, and it has been rather interesting to follow through the decades that the attitudes have

---

[138] For the history of ISRHML, see www.isrhml.org.umu.se/. Bibliographies can be found under Publications (visited 8 June 2008).

[139] See www.isrhml.org.umu.se/publications/, published monographs of the society's past meetings (visited 9 January 2009).

[140] Medline is the US National Library of Medicine's premier bibliographic database and is the largest component of PubMed; see www.ncbi.nlm.nih.gov/sites/entrez?db=pubmed (visited 26 November 2008).

totally changed and I think this is in parallel with the advancement of women in societies.

O'Leary: We have been looking at various different branches of science and the effects that they have had or not had on breastfeeding practice in society and on the wards. But there is one branch of science that we have omitted, which is the science of marketing, and that's a science which has developed in width, breadth and depth in the last 20 or 30 years in an incredible way. Our mothers and grandmothers were not brand-aware in the way that we are and our children are. Marketing has taken on a wider significance than just advertising. There have been instances of marketing personnel helping to train health professionals and this must have some effect on what is found, what is thought to be normal, what is just considered the usual thing that people do. Of course it has an influence on the mothers as well. You only have to walk into a supermarket to see the usual way of feeding a baby. You see it all around, the equipment and gadgets and the things on display as well as the milk. So I think this social science of marketing has probably been more influential than any of our efforts, unfortunately, to tell the truth about the value of breastfeeding and breast-milk.

Woolridge: One thing that has been clear is that the rules that are entrenched within Baby Friendly hospitals were in existence and being practised in this country long before that. Because certainly one thing the COMA report did do was to set down building blocks by entrenching demand feeding, and uninterrupted contact between the mother and baby. The nice thing about the OPCS and ONS reports is that not only did they document changes in the rate but also changes in practice.[141] These incremental changes in practice coincided with the changes in the rate. One thing I have never been clear on is whether they have actually driven the changes in practice, or whether they created an atmosphere which reflected what was naturally happening.

I think something that is relevant to what Rachel has just said is that the very first hospital to put itself forward for accreditation as Baby Friendly was very much a guinea pig. Cynthia Rickett put forward Sunderland District General Hospital to be evaluated and because we were unused to the process we had a midwife from Sweden, Anna-Berit Ransjö-Arvidson, come over to help make sure we were doing things properly. When she walked on to the wards at a British hospital she came across, for the first time in her life, 'ready-to-feed'

---

[141] See note 16.

bottles of formula. Little tiny baby bottles, which she found captivating and wanted to take back purely for their interest value.[142] This part of the commercial promotion of formula is also found to be a very attractive vehicle in which to make formulae available for hospitals, both practical and convenient, and very attractive for mothers to use. I think there is an important issue in looking at the commercial influence in hospitals as to whether it was an unavoidable conducive element for mothers.

Dr Mary Smale: I'm a National Childbirth Trust breastfeeding counsellor. I am taking up the issue of branding. I was told from a very young age by my bottle-feeding mother that I was given Cow and Gate in 1943 because that was what the Queen was given. The young princesses were fed on this, which was far superior, of course, to National Dried Milk and which was what we as a middle class family could afford.[143]

I think maybe if we did lots and lots of oral history on this we'd find the meanings of all sorts of things that would be very interesting. I would also like to ask a question. Who owns time? And the other thing is why the changes may be happening? To give you a small example: before I moved to the south of England I spent 30 years in the Humberside area, and in north Hull the starting rate for breastfeeding in one area was 14 per cent. After the peer support training scheme that I taught we had a report back from a mother who said she had asked someone whether they were going to breastfeed and this young mum said: 'Yeah, it's dead trendy now.'[144]

Weaver: Shall we go back to the early days again and to some of the official reports? Thinking about that; there was the present-day practice document in 1974. John, can you tell us a little bit about that?

Mr John Wells: I think I am one of the monkeys in the barrel that was referred to previously.[145] I am a paediatric nutritionist and I came into industry in the

---

[142] The Symons collection in the museum of the Royal College of Physicians contains a collection of infant feeding cups, as well as nipple shields. See www.rcplondon.ac.uk/heritage/medicalInstruments/ (visited 23 October 2008).

[143] See note 110.

[144] Dr Mary Smale wrote: 'A peer support training scheme was delivered by me as an NCT breastfeeding counsellor funded by North Hull Surestart to local women in early 2001.' E-mail to Mrs Lois Reynolds, 29 October 2008.

[145] See page 55.

late 1960s and focused on paediatric nutrition with Cow and Gate and latterly Nutricia. It's very clear to me when I joined the company that the first *Present-Day Practice in Infant Feeding* report had a very dramatic impact on the way industry was being viewed and that the products had many shortcomings in terms of their composition.[146] Some of these have been referred to in terms of too high solutes, particularly sodium, high phosphate, the use of sugar in reconstituting feeds and very complex making-up instructions, which mothers found difficult to follow and as a result invariably had a tendency to over-concentrate. There were a number of common problems that were found at the time and seen by paediatricians, such as dehydration, hypernatraemia, hypocalcaemic tetany and infantile obesity, which were attributed to the use of formulae at that time.

It was clear that industry had to react to this. It's quite interesting to go back for just a moment to consider how this report actually originated, because although I wasn't at the meeting in Cambridge, my understanding was that the British Nutrition Foundation had a meeting on nutrition in Cambridge in the early 1970s where these problems in infants were being aired, particularly in relation to the shortcomings of infant formulae and the poor take-up of breastfeeding in the nation. And one or two of the industry members got up and said: 'Well, if the medical profession can tell us what to do, we will get on and do it.' It fell on the then Department of Health and Social Security to convene a panel on child nutrition and from that emerged the first *Present-Day Practice in Infant Feeding* report.[147] So I think that was a very important outcome of the meeting of the British Nutrition Foundation in Cambridge.

Once the shortcomings were confirmed in a COMA grey report, industry got full cooperation with the paediatric profession, particularly the paediatricians, to sort out these irregularities in composition so that by the early 1980s when I became involved in the science of infant formulae, these were, in fact, resolved. This led to a very competitive communication to health professionals in infant formula brochures about whose formula was closest to breast-milk [see Figures 12 and 13]. In those days the comparisons were rather at a ridiculous level, where 1–2 milligrams of sodium per decilitre were considered to be superior if they were lower and closer to human milk composition than in another brand. But in fact it would appear at that time that health professionals did actually

---

[146] Oppé *et al.* (1974). See also DHSS (1977); Macy *et al.* (1953).

[147] DHSS COMA Working Party on the Composition of Foods for Infants and Young Children. Professor Thomas Oppé was the chairman.

COMPARISON OF THE COMPOSITION OF BREASTMILK, COWS' MILK
AND TWO INFANT MILK FORMULAS AVAILABLE IN 1974 (per 100ml)

		Breast Milk	Cows' Milk	Cow & Gate Babymilk 1*	National Dried Full Cream*
Major Nutrients					
Protein	g	1.2	3.3	2.4	2.5
Fat	g	3.8	3.7	1.9	2.4
Carbohydrate	g	7.0	4.8	7.0	5.9†
Minerals					
Calcium	mg	33	125	84	83
Phosphorus	mg	15	96	65	67
Sodium	mg	15	58	41	40
Potassium	mg	55	138	104	109
Chloride	mg	43	103	ns	ns
Magnesium	mg	4	12	8.9	10.2
Iron	mg	0.15	0.1	0.5	0.48
Zinc	mg	0.5	0.4	0.2	ns
Copper	µg	40	30	12.6	ns
Vitamins					
A Retinol	µg	58	40	100	23
D₃ Cholecalciferol	µg	0.01	0.06	1.1	0.8
C Ascorbic Acid	mg	4.3	1.6	3.5	2.4
Energy					
	kcal	67	66	54	55†

ns   Not stated
*   No longer manufactured
†   Includes sugar added in accordance with instructions

Source: Present Day Practice in Infant Feeding (1974)

Figure 12: Comparison of the composition of cows' milk with infant formula
in 1974. Source: Cow and Gate (1989).

COMPOSITION OF MATURE HUMAN MILK AND TYPICAL CURRENT
DAY INFANT FORMULAS COMPARED WITH DHSS GUIDELINES (per 100ml)

		Mature Breastmilk Mean	Range	DHSS Guidelines	Cow & Gate Premium	Cow & Gate Plus
Major Nutrients						
Protein	g	1.3	1.2–1.4	1.2–2.0*	1.5	1.9
Fat	g	4.2	3.7–4.8	2.3–5.0	3.6	3.4
Lactose	g	7.4	7.1–7.8	2.5–8.0	7.3	7.3
Minerals						
Calcium	mg	35	32–36	30–120	54	85
Phosphorus	mg	15	14–15	15–60	27	55
Sodium	mg	15	11–20	15–35	18	25
Potassium	mg	60	57–62	50–100	65	100
Chloride	mg	43	35–55	40–80	40	60
Magnesium	mg	2.8	2.6–3.0	2.8–12	5	7
Iron	µg	76	62–93	70–700	500	500
Zinc	µg	295	260–330	200–600**	400	400
Iodine	µg	7	2–12	ns	7	7
Manganese	µg	ns	ns	ns	7	7
Copper	µg	39	37–43	10–60**	40	40
Vitamins						
A Retinol	µg	60	40–76	40–150	80	80
D₃ Cholecalciferol	µg	ns	ns	0.7–1.3	1.1	1.1
E dl-α-Tocopherol	mg	0.35	0.29–0.39	0.3–ns	1.1	1.1
K₁ Phytomenadione	µg	ns	ns	1.5–ns	5	5
B₁ Thiamin	µg	16	13–21	13–ns	40	40
B₂ Riboflavin	µg	31	31	30–ns	100	100
B₆ Pyridoxine	µg	5.9	5.1–7.2	5–ns	40	40
B₁₂ Cyanocobalamin	µg	0.01	0.01	0.01–ns	0.2	0.2
Nicotinic Acid	µg	230	210–270	230–ns	400	400
Pantothenic Acid	µg	260	220–330	200–ns	300	300
Biotin	µg	0.76	0.52–1.13	0.5–ns	1.5	1.5
Folic Acid	µg	5.2	3.1–6.2	3–ns	10	10
C Ascorbic Acid	mg	3.8	3.1–4.5	3–ns	8	8
Energy						
	kJ	293	270–315	270–315	275	275
	kcal	70	65–75	65–75	66	66

* Protein having a casein:whey ratio similar to breastmilk
** Tentative guideline

Sources: The Composition of Mature Human Milk (1977)
         Artificial Feeds for the Young Infant (1980)
         Cow & Gate data

Figure 13: Comparison of the composition of human milk with infant formula in
the early 1980s. Source: Cow and Gate (1989).

make or base some of their recommendations on these types of comparisons, and the industry fed them this sort of information.

During the 1980s and 1990s, of course, as the call for mothers to breastfeed strengthened, the whole issue became much more politicized and the industry through the offices of the UK Food and Drink Federation set up a forum called the Infant and Dietetic Food Association. There the views of industry were collected and used, in a way, to explain the industry viewpoint on the various issues of the day.[148] This would involve responding to government reports, to proposed legislation, and other issues such as the distribution of literature. Also, at that time it was becoming clear that the employees of the infant formulae companies were finding it more difficult to communicate changes in infant formulae to health professionals. It was more difficult for representatives to access maternity wards and neonatal units, paediatricians were less available for discussion on infant nutrition issues. There was either a lessening or an absence of instruction on the preparation of infant formulae to mothers in antenatal clinics. And there was an attitude that was picked up that advances in infant formula design, which brought it closer to human milk, were in some way resented by some health professionals, because this diminished the superiority of human milk.

Lastly, one of the consequences of having reduced access to the medical profession was that it was more difficult to carry out legitimate studies that had been through proper ethics committees and so on, and this was partly due to the fact that nursing staff were particularly concerned that if a mother was seen to be participating in a study, getting study formula which would be free of charge, then this could negatively influence breastfeeding mothers, or some nurses just did not want to cooperate or be seen to be cooperating with an infant formula company. So these are some of the situations that arose during my time with Nutricia.[149]

Weaver: There may be some reaction to that, but I also want to talk about the other important reports in a minute.

Akre: We are not going to have time to do anything about it this evening, but I want to suggest building on what the last speaker said by asking how we are going to move infant formula, which started out as an emergency nutrition

---

[148] See www.idfa.org.uk/about.aspx (visited 7 August 2008).

[149] Nutricia Ltd has been part of the Danone Group of companies since 2007. It specializes in developing and manufacturing infant milk formula and nutritional supplements for medicinal use.

intervention, from the kitchen pantry back into the medicine cabinet or first aid kit, where it got its start. That is the challenge we face.

We talk a lot about morbidity and mortality, and prevalence and duration of breastfeeding in developing countries and so-called developed countries. That's not a bad place to start the conversation, but I think we need to project, individually and collectively, how we want the next generation to proceed. All governments are commercial-interest friendly, by definition, for a variety of reasons, including employment creation, improved balance of payments, income generation, all sorts of things. So, how are we going to convince governments that it is in their best interest, in the short and longer term, to promote nature's food, not just as a way of feeding today's babies, but having an impact on health throughout the life course, not only of babies, but of today's and tomorrow's mothers as well.

Smale: I am very aware of a huge paradox here. You want to go from the pantry to the medicine cupboard, yes? But in doing that you actually cut lots of people out and I would say today that the main group who have been left out are the mothers.[150] I have to say that today's meeting has been progressed by a largely masculine-led group, and if you go from the pantry to the medicine cupboard you gain some things and you lose some things, and that needs looking at. It can be looked at historically; if you look at Jacqueline Wolf's description of the pathologization of breastfeeding you will see that almost every discovery in breastfeeding has unfortunately then become pathologized.[151] You only have to identify 'let down' or 'ejection reflex' to find, amazingly, it doesn't work, but it frighteningly and alarmingly disappears under any sort of stress, which I am afraid is nonsense, isn't it? Women in the audience who have been breastfeeding mothers have been quite upset from time to time, but amazingly, astonishingly, mothers managed to continue to breastfeed in spite of this. And it is frightening to be told that it's their anxiety that's frightening away their breastfeeding. And then if we talk about the foremilk/hindmilk divide, if there is such a thing, which there isn't – thank goodness for Mike's research – it's a graduation thing, but if we talk about that we suddenly get a whole host of mothers ringing up saying they are frightened to death about not giving the baby enough hindmilk. How long should I be letting him stay on to get to the hindmilk? So what we do is we pathologize. We have a huge paradox.

---

[150] Dr Mary Smale wrote: 'My main concern is that today's discussion mainly, though not exclusively, portrays women as "acted upon", while scientific careers were forged elsewhere, defining terms, rather than listening to women.' Note on draft transcript, 7 September 2007.

[151] Wolf (2001).

Weaver: That's a very clear point. There's a bit of pathology that I would like to hear a bit about that I think is from a different category and that's Peter Howie's work and the public health impact of their studies that reinforced the value of breast-milk.

Howie: When I went to Dundee, one day I was approached by a student midwife who wanted to do a project on the benefits of breastfeeding. She asked if I could provide information that showed that breastfeeding was healthier for the baby. I thought about it, and then went to the literature, and actually it was quite difficult to find – this was in 1984. In fact, just then there had been a publication by Howard Bauchner and his colleagues from the US, which had reviewed all the articles in the English language literature between 1970 and 1984, which had the objective of looking at the relationship between breastfeeding and prevention of infectious disease, especially diarrhoeal and respiratory disease.[152] They looked at all the papers and applied four methodological criteria to evaluate the robustness of the studies: (i) whether the studies had defined what they meant by full, partial, or token breastfeeding; (ii) whether they defined what was meant by illness; (iii) whether they had a study that made sure that observer bias didn't distort the results; and, most importantly, (iv) that they had taken into account the confounding variables, particularly social class, or whether there was another, older child in the family. After they applied these four criteria to all the studies they found that every one of them, bar two, was deficient methodologically; and the two that were thought to be methodologically OK had sample sizes of only 40 and 60 patients respectively. When we looked at it, we thought that the minimal sample size for a satisfactory study was 560. We thought that even these two studies were methodologically unsound. It came to the point that everyone was saying, 'breast is best', and there was actually no sound evidence to back that up.

Now, I think that shows that it's very wrong to have study after study which is methodologically unsound, and that was a major problem for breastfeeding. We thought that what was needed was a study that met the methodological criteria set down by Bauchner and colleagues and that's what we did. I recruited Stewart Forsyth, who can't be here today, to give us paediatric expertise, and Charles Florey, an epidemiologist, to make sure that the construction of the study and the statistics were done properly.[153] When we did the study in view of what Bauchner had found, I thought we would find trivial differences, but

---

[152] Bauchner *et al.* (1986).

[153] See, for example, Anderson *et al.* (2001); Alder *et al.* (2004).

in point of fact we found, comparing women who had been breastfeeding for 13 weeks against women who had bottle-fed right from the start, that there was an eightfold difference in significant diarrhoeal disease and hospital admission. If you *then* allowed for confounding variables, the difference narrowed to fivefold; still a huge difference. We came to the conclusion that this showed very strong evidence that breastfeeding did make a difference in a country such as our own.

It's quite interesting that *Pediatrics,* of three weeks ago, carried a publication showing (somewhat 'surprisingly,' it says) that breastfeeding reduces diarrhoeal and respiratory infection.[154] This paper in *Pediatrics* may be of great interest to the people here today, particularly those who are promoting breastfeeding: it is the UK millennium cohort study, published by Maria Quigley, Yvonne Kelly and Amanda Sacker from the national perinatal epidemiology unit in Oxford and the department of epidemiology and public health at UCL. The sample size is almost 16 000 and it says that full prolonged breastfeeding reduces hospital admissions for diarrhoeal disease by 50 per cent and respiratory infections by 27 per cent, and the conclusion, if I could just read out:

> Our findings confirm that breastfeeding, particularly when exclusive and prolonged, protects against severe morbidity in contemporary UK. In our study, only 1.2 per cent of infants were exclusively breastfed for at least six months, and the protective effects of breastfeeding were large; a population-level increase in exclusive, prolonged breastfeeding would be of great public health benefit.[155]

Now they happily refer to our paper and the findings are exactly comparable.[156] I think it was James Akre who said: 'Can we bring a lever on public health policy?' To my mind, this might well be the lever. This is a large study, saying that universal breastfeeding would have a major impact on infant health.

Weaver: This is an example of the Americans not wanting to read the European literature, isn't it?

---

[154] Quigley *et al.* (2007).

[155] Quigley *et al.* (2007): 841. The study included 15 890 healthy, singleton, full-term infants who were born in 2000–02. See also Smith and Joshi (2002); Plewis (2004). Further details available at www.data-archive. ac.uk/findingdata/snDescription.asp?sn=4683&key=Millennium+Cohort+Study (visited 18 June 2008).

[156] Howie *et al.* (1990).

Howie: This is in *Pediatrics,* the journal of the American Academy of Pediatrics, of 4 April 2007.

Weaver: Peter's work gave evidence and support for some of the recommendations of your report, Forrester Cockburn, in 1994, which was quite an important document, I think.

Cockburn: The report was *Weaning and the Weaning Diet.*[157] You asked me earlier how it came about. Mainly it came about because of the health visitors at the clinic I used to do on Friday afternoons at Drumchapel, who said: 'We need clear guidance.' I replied: 'You know more about weaning than I do.' I didn't want to take on this topic of weaning and the weaning diet, because I knew it had many pitfalls. At the time I was chairman of the panel on child nutrition of COMA, following on after Tom Oppé.[158] Quite a few people in this room today were on that committee – midwives, scientists of various sorts, paediatricians – joined me to produce that report under the eagle eye of the late Petra Clarke. We wanted to emphasize that weaning was not stopping breastfeeding; weaning was introducing new elements of diet at the right time to a breastfeeding infant. We did not wish midwives and others to think that weaning was stopping breastfeeding. Just as breast-milk protects against infections, as Peter was saying, it also protects against some of the foodstuffs that perhaps are not always the best thing for infants. It's important that breast-milk and the new food substances that are being introduced are given together for some time. So we looked not just at weaning and weaning foods; we looked at the whole process of weaning, and tried to come up with some guidance. But, I think the thing we wanted to emphasize was that weaning was not stopping breastfeeding, but the introduction of other elements of diet which are important to bottle and breastfed infants as they get bigger and require different foods.

Weaver: Was this influential and did it affect midwives?

Dr Penny Stanway: I wrote *Breast is Best* in 1978 as a handbook for mothers, because I had been working in community paediatrics and was appalled at what was taught about breastfeeding.[159] May I make a big plea for the full half-hour to discuss mother-to-mother support groups, please? The allotted 30 minutes looks like being 25 minutes short, and going with that would be a great pity and

---

[157] DoH (1994).

[158] See page 70 and note 108.

[159] Stanway and Stanway (1978).

reflect a lack of recognition of the balance of contributions to the resurgence of breastfeeding.[160]

I'd like to point out that breastfeeding – which incidentally should be all one word, not hyphenated – is a physiological process that relies on mother–baby and baby–mother interactions. It also has heaps of non-medical benefits not just to babies and mothers, but also to fathers and society as a whole. And it's terribly important not to over-medicalize it.

Today's discussions have been very interesting but very medical, and I feel annoyed that over-runs on the timing of several discussions may stop us giving fair consideration to the vital contributions of mother-to-mother groups. These embody a growing base of experience, skills and knowledge about how women can empower, encourage and support each other while making choices and learning how to breastfeed successfully, and how men can help. So, may I repeat my plea for adequate time for them?

Alder: Not just self-help groups. I am a psychologist and I think the psychological aspect is hugely important. Now, I think that there were more influences. My research was in Edinburgh in the 1970s and the 1980s; demand feeding was becoming much more popular. Once you remove that time constraint, mothers are then exposed to their babies – demand means demand – so the babies make demands on the mothers. Therefore we have a consequence for the mothers. One of the consequences is increased fatigue, breastfed babies wake more often in the night and for longer. So, this is a considerable demand. Without social support, without support groups, it is very difficult. I think one of the consequences of the medical research and the demand feeding, and it was all worked out physiologically, is that you have then got a different social situation for the mother. I was looking particularly at sexuality, and at the MRC reproductive biology unit I was supposed to be looking at hormone effects of sexuality in the postnatal period, which is very important for mothers and for couples. I found that fatigue was much more important. I think it is possible then that the increase in numbers of mothers breastfeeding was a result of the support groups, because the mothers needed support. You can't have a mother in our society breastfeeding on demand, frequently, exclusively, with nobody else doing it,

---

[160] A general draft outline of each Witness Seminar is circulated among all participants prior to the meeting. The specific timings given on the outline are flexible and on this occasion a number of the earlier topics were discussed for longer than anticipated so that not all of the issues listed could be covered in the same depth. We hope that even an inadequate discussion will signal their importance for future study. See Appendix 2 for the chairman's reflection on this issue.

because it's not that easy to express often. So I think the support groups could have been extremely influential. Maybe that's why there was a lag, and I would like Jenny Warren to come in and say why we are now getting some increase.

Warren: I do want to join in. I am rather disappointed that we have concentrated a lot on the medical side as well. But I would acknowledge that a lot of the papers that have been published and documents written have allowed many of us to engage with the powers that be to try to establish support for breastfeeding. We have mentioned the Joint Breastfeeding Initiative which is where Edwina Currie challenged the health professionals and the voluntary organizations to get together and support breastfeeding together and I think it was crucially important that that happened throughout the UK.[161] In Scotland we certainly went on from the concept of the Joint Breastfeeding Initiative; it was a multidisciplinary input and mothers were on these groups. We moved on to a strategic approach. We included the Baby Friendly Initiative in that strategic approach. But we did have this multifaceted approach and we had strategy groups all over Scotland, who were implementing strategy broadly based on the breastfeeding in Scotland paper written by Campbell and Jones in 1994.[162] So a lot of the good work was done in Scotland and was achieved through cooperation and real commitment and enthusiasm rather than through financial support from government. I would be disappointed if that's not acknowledged in *The Resurgence of Breastfeeding* (this volume).

Weaver: We want to hear what happened.

Miss Carol Williams: I think my point follows on quite nicely from Jenny Warren. I felt we needed also to acknowledge that although we have had lots of discussion on the science involved, if we actually look back since 1975, I think breastfeeding support is evident as being almost like a Cinderella service. There's been very scant commitment of resources and we know that we have studies that prove that mother-to-mother support is often the most effective, but I think that it's been used as a kind of get-out clause for not actually putting money there. I have had situations locally where if one of my peer supporters does Reiki healing with women in deprived areas, they can be paid £40 an hour, but if they go to do breastfeeding support, it has got to be voluntary. It's just ridiculous and I really question, when we talk about resurgence of breastfeeding, whether we have got a resurgence of policy commitment. Again, if you look back historically I think

---

[161] See note 105.

[162] Campbell and Jones (1994). See also Britten and McInnes (1999).

it's quite useful to bear in mind that for 35 years we had National Dried Milk, and my understanding is that when National Dried Milk finally disappeared in 1976, it was more to do with concern about unfair competition with the milk companies than any kind of conviction that it wasn't a good idea in itself. If we come to today and this alleged resurgence of interest (if it is interest) in breastfeeding, is it because of the connection with obesity? Somewhere along the line the fact that breastfeeding is good in its own right has not been enough. And historically, that question has been there all the way through.

Mrs Jill Dye: I am from the La Leche League so I do want to talk about breastfeeding support groups. You can breastfeed without a support group; it is possible to do it. It was Penny Stanway's book that actually helped me the most with my first two children because I read that it was OK, not that I had to, but OK to exclusively feed for six months, and OK to breastfeed for two years.[163] So that got me through. With my third I had tremendous problems, it was not the milk; I didn't think I had any milk, but I wanted to breastfeed him. It was a voluntary group, and I thought: 'They can help me feed my baby at the breast even if I don't have any milk.' So I got the: 'You are going to be able to do it, you are going to get the milk, it's going to happen.' Wonderful. It did. I kept on going to the group and I am still involved. But it was wonderful. We help hundreds of mothers. I probably help, personally, several hundreds of mothers a year and I find it's an incredible burden in a way because it's all down to me and women like me trying to do this and we are but a drop in the ocean. We cannot do it by ourselves. We should all be working together to normalize breastfeeding, which is what did not happen in the 1980s when we tried to get together. I was on the Joint Breastfeeding Initiative executive group. Rachel O'Leary was on that and there are other people in this room who were in that group as well. We all tried to work very hard together. I can remember Tony Williams saying: 'We have to stop talking about making women feel guilty and start telling them the truth.' This was in 1989, I think, and we have been trying all this time. A very important thing is that if there is anything to do with the resurgence of breastfeeding we have been working together, but it doesn't seem to have changed. Here we are, 30 years later, and it has not changed.

Weaver: I hoped we would concentrate on the question, towards the end, whether or not there has been a resurgence of breastfeeding?

Ms Hilary English: I am a National Childbirth Trust breastfeeding counsellor and tutor; I have been on Royal College of Midwives working parties to help

---

[163] Stanway and Stanway (1978).

with breastfeeding and a lactation consultant, etc. and I am a volunteer. Mostly I am a volunteer. I support a lot of women and hopefully I pick up some of the pieces that the health professionals, with great respect, leave behind. I wanted to pick up on Carol Williams's point about the respect that is given to breastfeeding. At the moment, breastfeeding is being looked after in my area by auxiliaries because the midwives are too busy. There is not enough time for a midwife to help with breastfeeding. Not even to get a baby attached, let alone to stay through one feed. This is being left to auxiliary staff who are low-paid workers. Breastfeeding status is absolutely minimal and until this is corrected and the value of breastfeeding, the health value, even the economic value and medical value, whatever, is given some recognition we will not get anywhere.

Palmer: I'm a nutritionist at the London School of Hygiene and Tropical Medicine but I'm interested in the social, political and human side of this subject. I keep hearing: 'How can we persuade?' Or: 'Why doesn't the NHS do and such and such?' I don't think we need to persuade or promote but to remove the enormous constraints on breastfeeding. Social and cultural influences are powerful. When I worked in Mozambique in the early 1980s, UNICEF were providing infant formula in bottles which were lethal, yet that was the state of UNICEF's awareness at that time.[164] Later UNICEF became a leading advocate for control of such harmful distribution. I am saying this to illustrate that the idea that women as individuals choose their feeding method is false. Only educated women in Mozambique ever dreamed of bottle-feeding, whereas in the UK these are the women who want to breastfeed. This decision is often influenced artificially through the pressures of vested interests.

I am interested to see an industry representative here today. One of my students did an investigation of infant feeding product promotion in popular parents' magazines for her dissertation. The editorial followed along a culture of branded-product loyalty focused on pregnant women and new parents. Miriam Stoppard

---

[164] Ms Gabrielle Palmer wrote: 'Artificial feeding has at least a sixfold mortality risk. See WHO Collaborative Study Team (2000) on the role of breastfeeding in the prevention of infant mortality. The link between artificial feeding and high mortality was documented throughout the twentieth century, especially in developing countries [Scrimshaw *et al.* (1968)]. I was working in Mozambique between 1981 and 1983 and by then there was substantial literature and widespread international media coverage of the lethal effects of artificial feeding. Chetley (1979) has a 280-article bibliography on the topic. In 1980 Papua New Guinea had already introduced legislation to restrict the sale of feeding bottles there [Biddulph (1980)]. My point is that it was an embarrassment for UNICEF to have displayed such lack of awareness.' E-mail to Ms Stefania Crowther, 1 December 2008.

wrote an editorial that echoed the marketing. It is the little points that are so insidious, such as: 'You won't want to feed your baby on demand all the time.'[165]

Also there has been a move that has been led by the commercial promotion of breast pumps. I was interested in Roger Short's information about women feeding 98 times a day. This contrasts with the trend, certainly in the US and more and more so here, that breastfeeding equates with pumping breast-milk. Of course it doesn't. In the US, six million breast pumps are sold each year. That is one and a half breast pumps per baby. That is not breastfeeding: the baby does not have the psychological warmth, it's not having the skin contact, which changes both the mother's and baby's hormones. It's making money all the time. Certainly in this country if you read all the magazines, they present a lifestyle that is not conducive to breastfeeding. Maybe a little bit, but mostly they promote pumping and getting your husband to give pumped breast-milk in a bottle at night. We are all victims of it. We are leaving this out and behaving as though people do what is said in the *Lancet*. People don't do what they say in the *Lancet*; people do what *Vogue* tells them to do, or *Cosmo*, or *Parents and Babies*. I think we are forgetting a big pressure that changes us much more powerfully and subtly than any of the good scientific evidence.

Weaver: We have just touched on this subject, but it is a very complex and wide one. I think we have heard about many dimensions of the whole topic. There's no way that I can summarize, nor is it appropriate for me to do so, but I am going to ask Mary Renfrew to wind up.

Renfrew: I am not going to attempt to summarize, but I do want to take another few minutes to expand the discussion. I completely agree with Penny's statement a minute ago about the fundamental importance of support groups. I just want to take a few minutes to focus on what I think the biggest problems are here, and therefore why women as women and women working together are a huge part of the emphasis and have been over the last 25 years. We are facing a very strange culture in this country, where, in a study that I did a few years ago with Mike Woolridge, teenagers told us that, yes, they felt that the right thing to do was breastfeed their babies, but they actually thought the act of breastfeeding was immoral, to expose a breast in public was something that was wrong and perverted, and to be seen to be was perverted. Now, if we take that as a starting point – the very bizarre society that we live in in the UK – what I have seen, working with and experiencing the National Childbirth Trust, La Leche League,

---

[165] See Wake (2006).

the Breastfeeding Network and the Association of Breastfeeding Mothers, over the last 25–30 years, has been a huge force for good trying hard to counter those societal forces so that women can do what women are, in part, born to do. They are born to do many other things too, but one of them is breastfeed the baby. The impact of the support groups on women's lives and indeed on the psyche of the health service, among others has been fundamentally important and I would hate to think that this history today is going to miss that.

We have heard lots of bits through the day, people have interjected, but to try to pull that together: support groups have been important in educating health professionals, they have been important to training counsellors – thousands of them, leaders and counsellors across the country today, supporting tens of thousands of women, millions over the years – when the health service had abandoned them, and that was all that they had. They have informed policy, they are increasingly being built into policy decisions and included in consultations on policies at a national level and indeed at international level. They have informed research, and, in my own experience, actually participated in research. I think we ran the first ever randomized controlled trial in which women were randomized by a consumer support group and took part in the trial and were followed up by a consumer support group; the first example of a randomized trial by a lay group, the National Childbirth Trust.[166] In peer reviewing research, the most astute comments I ever get from any of my research reports are always from my consumer support group colleagues, who have been incredibly valuable.[167] The Cochrane reviews, the NICE reports and so on, the Department of Health reports, over the years, I have learned from support groups to keep women at the heart of everything; they do it all the time and they have done it brilliantly today, although not as much as we could have. They are sitting right in the middle of everything. Women's experiences, women's feelings, women's real lived experiences, reflected against or beside the realities of research, and that's always important. They also have this tremendous commitment to the evidence base, to the accuracy of information, making sure that whatever happens does not harm and does good, and in my whole experience they have been absolutely radical about that. They have been proponents of peer support from the very, very earliest period of La Leche League peer support schemes and through into the much, much bigger, National Childbirth Trust and Breastfeeding Network peer support groups, which in my experience are now reaching the poorest part

---

[166] The MAIN Trial Collaborative Group (1994); Renfrew and McCandlish (1992).

[167] Allain and Kean (2007). See www.ibfan.org (visited 11 August 2008).

of this country in the way that the health service is struggling to do. Find a Baby Café somewhere in a very poor multiethnic part of an urban conglomeration and there you will find a support group, with trained peer supporters, and they are making that happen fantastically. There are people in this room who have been hugely instrumental in that. That's where we are going to make the difference. The resistance rates have been in the youngest, the poorest, the white communities in this country, and that's where the difference is going to come. I think we are about to see a resurgence of breastfeeding because a lot of the pieces are now in place in policy terms and the support groups working hand-in-hand with the health service are there. They were ahead of the health service all the way. They have retained local roots, these national organizations, in forming policy, local routes right down to the breastfeeding women.

We can all learn advocacy also from the support groups, who are fighting, going out to support real women when they have been put out of restaurants and told not to breastfeed in public, and we need all the support groups to make sure that doesn't continue to happen. They have been linked in with the overall philosophy of natural childbearing, which I think is a hugely important issue that we have touched on today in part, but it's very important and needs more discussion. I really notice the difference when I go to countries that don't have support groups. I have done a lot of work in the Netherlands and some in Germany, for example, where there is no tradition of support groups. They don't know how to create change, and if we ask Elisabet Helsing about mother-to-mother groups in Norway, that's how they did it there and I absolutely agree: that's how we are going to do it here. The support groups have been fed by the science and they have taken it up and they have championed it (and that's where the links are and that's where I think that happens). We can do whatever we like in our research studies, nothing is going to happen unless women and their supporting men get out there and actually make those changes happen at policy level, at practice level and in women's own homes, on the streets, in the shops and on the buses, where women need to be feeding their babies and travelling.

Just one thing to mention, one of the things that we identified when we did our work for NICE over the last couple of years and produced a report.[168] The response to the evidence-based review and the national consultation that we carried out to do that was incredibly strong and it said that in order to make all the kinds of changes that are needed, first of all you have got to create change in

---

[168] NICE (2008). See also Renfrew and Hall (2008).

society. You have got to educate children, you have got to help women combine work and breastfeeding. You have got to have a national strategy to lead it and make sure it reaches all the parts across government. You have got to facilitate breastfeeding in public and so on. I am smiling at Jenny because they have done so much of this in Scotland already. But that was what our work said. Now in fact NICE wouldn't act on that, because it's not mandated to that societal level, it can only at the moment speak to the health service, but those recommendations have been taken up by a new group called the Breastfeeding Manifesto Coalition which is a coalition of all the support groups, with all the Royal Colleges, with other groups like UNISON and other organizations that have come together under the leadership of an amazing woman called Alison Baum, who happens to be David Baum's niece, which is an interesting circle here. She comes from a support group background and not from a health professional background, and has tied together over 30 organizations, who have already met with the public health minister, who have already got MPs in to talk to Tony Blair, they have already got Gordon Brown standing up and talking about this organization at policy level. I am hugely inspired by that, and that organization is dedicated to addressing inequalities in health and tackling the problems of breastfeeding in the communities where the rates are lowest, which is what I think we should be doing for the next 25 years, bringing to bear all the evidence-based strategies we now know work, funding them properly, making them happen and using the policy doors which are currently open. Working together as the support groups have modelled for years, working together with each other and working together with health professionals and anybody who would work with them to create real change for women and I want that to be the legacy of the support groups: to remember that we are talking about women and babies.

Weaver: Roger wants to say something before we close.

Short: I think we know enough to insist that there should be a health warning on every packet of infant formula sold in Britain or anywhere else in the world.

Weaver: The time is up. Clearly this is a very broad, interesting subject and I think it will be the historians in another 50 years who will have to look back and say whether we were talking about a resurgence of breastfeeding, the beginning, the middle, the end, and what we mean about resurgence of breastfeeding. But I am very grateful to everyone who has come. Daphne will be in touch with us all about the proceedings of this meeting and I hope everyone will be happy to contribute and edit their contributions and so on.

Howie: I am sure I speak for everybody here when I thank the History of Twentieth Century Medicine Group of the Wellcome Trust Centre for setting up this meeting. I was delighted to see that they have thought that this was one of the priorities amongst all the possibilities that come forward, and I think they deserve enormous credit and thanks for doing so.

Dr Daphne Christie: Unfortunately, Dr Tansey has had to leave the meeting early, and therefore on behalf of the Wellcome Trust Centre for the History of Medicine at UCL, I would like to thank you all for coming along and participating in today's seminar and to thank Professor Lawrence Weaver for his excellent chairing of the meeting.

Appendix 1

Recommended breastfeeding times as recorded in Mary Mayes' *Handbook of Midwifery*, 1937–80

Collated by Chloe Fisher

Mayes' Handbook of Midwifery[1]
1st edition 1937 Mary Mayes

1st day	5 minutes at each breast	8 hourly + boiled water
2nd day	7 minutes at each breast	6 hourly
3rd day	15 minutes at one breast	3 hourly
4th day	20 minutes at one breast	3 hourly

2nd edition, 1938, revised by Mrs M A Gannon

1st day	5 minutes at each breast	8 hourly + boiled water
2nd day	7 minutes at each breast	6 hourly
3rd day	15 minutes at one breast	3 hourly
4th day	20 minutes at one breast	3 hourly

3rd edition, 1941, revised by Mrs M A Gannon

1st day	5 minutes at each breast	8 hourly + boiled water
2nd day	7 minutes at each breast	6 hourly
3rd day	15 minutes at one breast	3 hourly
4th day	20 minutes at one breast	3 hourly

4th edition, 1953, revised by Mrs F D Thomas

1st day	2 minutes at each breast	8 hourly
2nd day	4 minutes at each breast	6 hourly
3rd day	6 minutes at each breast	4 hourly
4th day	8–10 minutes at each breast	4 hourly

5th edition, 1955, revised by Mrs F D Thomas

1st day	2 minutes at each breast	8 hourly
2nd day	4 minutes at each breast	6 hourly
3rd day	6 minutes at each breast	4 hourly
4th day	8–10 minutes at each breast	4 hourly

Mayes' Handbook for Midwives and Maternity Nurses

6th edition, 1959, revised by Mrs F D Thomas

1st day	2 minutes at each breast	8 hourly
2nd day	4 minutes at each breast	6 hourly
3rd day	6 minutes at each breast	4 hourly
4th day	8–10 minutes at each breast	4 hourly

7th edition, 1967, revised by Vera Da Cruz

1st day	2 minutes at each breast	8 hourly
2nd day	4 minutes at each breast	6 hourly
3rd day	6 minutes at each breast	4 hourly
4th day	8–10 minutes at each breast	4 hourly

Mayes' Midwifery: A Textbook for Midwives

8th edition, 1972, revised by Rosemary Bailey

1st day	2 minutes at each breast	8 hourly
2nd day	4 minutes at each breast	6 hourly
3rd day	6 minutes at each breast	4 hourly
4th day	8–10 minutes at each breast	4 hourly

9th edition, 1976, revised by Rosemary Bailey

1st day	2 minutes at each breast	8 hourly
2nd day	4 minutes at each breast	6 hourly
3rd day	6 minutes at each breast	4 hourly
4th day	8-10 minutes at each breast	4 hourly

10th edition, 1980, revised by Betty R Sweet

There should be no restriction on time at the breast.
The baby sucks until he is satisfied.
Complementary feeds should not be required.

Appendix 2

Resurgence of breastfeeding: metaphor and microcosm.
Chairman's reflections after the event

Lawrence Weaver, May 2007

The title of this Seminar – *The Resurgence of Breastfeeding* – implies a process occurring over time. In this respect the Witness Seminar differed from others that have focused on a discrete topic, such as a discovery, advance or innovation (ultrasound, peptic ulcer or genetic testing, for instance). Although a resurgence might properly be assumed to have a duration, a beginning and an end, an upward trajectory is its chief characteristic. In the event, the assumption that breastfeeding has been on the rise was called into question. Even if it were possible to trace an upturn in breastfeeding rates set in motion by changing maternal practices or professional attitudes, its trajectory has been far from linear. Participants representing different interests perceived the significance of 'key events' that might have powered the resurgence in very different ways. And, most significantly, there was a concern expressed by some that there has been no resurgence at all: a stasis in breastfeeding?

Nevertheless, the lack of unanimity about what 'happened' between 1975 and 2000 made for a lively debate. Starting with a survey of the science (or lack of it) thitherto underpinning rational advice about breastfeeding, an account of work done in the developing world generated shared memories by those involved, and led on to reflections by animal and human physiologists on their contributions, concentrating largely on the work of 'professionals'. As the seminar got going we heard from midwives and neonatologists, from national and international activists. As each spoke, the debate moved from recollection of what had happened to statements of what should have happened; voicing views more than involvement. This development reflected the nature of a topic that belongs to no single group exclusively (apart from mothers themselves). Although the interests of many participants overlapped, few were congruent. An example of this emerged with the parallel accounts of those involved in studying the nutritional contributions of breastfeeding to babies, and those interested in its contraceptive effects on mothers. These separate but parallel stories, even when they came together in WHO deliberations, were represented by separate people from different backgrounds.

The disjunction between the work of reproductive and lactational physiologists mirrored that between obstetricians and neonatologists, and between paediatricians and midwives, revealing a gender divide that might be said to begin and belong to the moment of birth. Those most intimately involved with the act of birth – mother and baby – are cared for by midwives and doctors, who if not both in attendance, certainly exercise control. Their strongest advocates, the breastfeeding support groups, articulated this view. Indeed, the powerlessness of mothers in a medical environment prompted a 'Foucaultian' view of how the medical gaze puts the event of 'birth' so firmly in the 'clinic'. The voices unrepresented were those of breastfeeding mothers themselves. There was a feeling that those concerned with supporting them were not 'heard' in a Witness Seminar chaired by a middle-aged professional man prone to concentrate on the science and official reports that presented themselves as handy milestones with which to steer the debate along an uncertain trajectory.

The meeting was both a metaphor and microcosm of how the subject of breastfeeding is seen by different groups, and the untidy discussion, which at times lost touch with events and tended to the polemical, reflected the real nature of the wider current debate. Indeed, the Seminar made it abundantly clear that breastfeeding is still a very live issue, and whether or not there has been a resurgence, its course has been far from straight, strong, upwards or fully run. Indeed, in the eyes of the support groups it has hardly begun. Nor was it clear what were the forces that had, or had not, driven the 'resurgence'. The focus on the science and policy behind breastfeeding promotion perhaps drowned the quieter voices of those closer to mothers and their concerns. The de-medicalization of childbirth, the support of mothers in hospital, the women's movement, were subjects hardly touched on in a Witness Seminar, which covered such a wide range and encompassed so many different groups. Some were left with a sense of frustration, even disappointment, about what did not happen, rather than what happened.

References

Abt A F, Garrison F H. (1965) *Abt-Garrison History of Pediatrics.* Philadelphia, PA: W D Saunders.

Alder E M, Williams F L, Anderson A S, Forsyth S, Florey Cdu V, Van der Velde P. (2004) What influences the timing of the introduction of solid food to infants? *British Journal of Nutrition* **92**: 527–31.

Allain A. (1981) WHO board endorses battle against bottle. *Development Forum* **9**: 15.

Allain A, Kean Y J. (2007) *Breaking the Rules: Stretching the rules 2007.* Penang, Malaysia: International Code Documentation Center.

Anand S K, Sandborg C, Robinson R G, Lieberman E. (1980) Neonatal hypernatraemia associated with elevated sodium concentration of breast-milk. *Journal of Paediatrics* **96**: 66–8.

Anderson A S, Guthrie C A, Alder E M, Forsyth S, Howie P W, Williams F L. (2001) Rattling the plate: reasons and rationales for early weaning. *Health Education Research* **16**: 471–9.

Anon. (1988) Lactational amenorrhea: experts recommend full breastfeeding as child spacing method. *Network* **10**: 12.

Apple R D. (1980) To be used only under the direction of a physician: commercial infant feeding and medical practice, 1870–1940. *Bulletin of the History of Medicine* **54**: 402–17.

Apple R D. (1986) Infant formula industry and pharmaceutical markets 1870–1910. *Journal of the History of Medicine* **41**: 3–23.

Apple R D. (1987) Mothers and Medicine: a social history of infant feeding, 1890–1950. Wisconsin Publications in the History of Science and Medicine no. 7. Madison, WI: University of Wisconsin Press.

Apple R D. (1994) The medicalization of infant feeding in the United States and New Zealand: two countries, one experience. *Journal of Human Lactation* **10**: 31–7.

Arneil G C, Creery R D G, Lloyud J K, Oppé T E, Stroud C E, Wharton B A, Widdowson E M. (1975) Letter: National Dried Milk. *Lancet* **i**: 450–1.

Baird D T. (1979) Endocrinology of female infertility. *British Medical Bulletin* **35**: 193–8.

Baker A A. (1956) Factory in a hospital. *Lancet* **270**: 278–9.

Bartington S, Griffiths L J, Tate A R, Dezateux C, Millennium Cohort Study Health Group. (2006) Are breastfeeding rates higher among mothers delivering in Baby Friendly accredited maternity units in the UK? *International Journal of Epidemiology* **35**: 1178–86.

Bauchner H, Leventhal J M, Shapiro E D. (1986) Studies of breastfeeding and infections: How good is the evidence? *Journal of the American Medical Association* **256**: 887–92.

Baum J D. (1979) Development of human milk banks. *Midwife, Health Visitor and Community Nurse* **15**: 126–31.

Baum J D, Harker P. (1975) Letter: National Dried Milk. *Lancet* **i**: 450.

Belton N R, Cockburn F, Forfar J O, Giles M M, Kirkwood J, Smith J, Thistlethwaite D, Turner T L, Wilkinson E M. (1977) Clinical and biochemical assessment of a modified evaporated milk for infant feeding. *Archives of Disease in Childhood* **52**: 167–75.

Benyamin Y S, Hassan M K. (1998) Feeding patterns in first two years of life in Basra, Iraq. *East Mediterranean Health Journal* **14**: 3.

Biddulph J. (1980) Impact of legislation restricting the sale of feeding bottles in Papua New Guinea. *Nutrition and Development* **3**: 4–8.

Bolling K, Grant C, Hamlyn B, Thornton A. (2007) *Infant Feeding Survey 2005*. London: The Information Centre for Health and Social Care. Freely available at www.ic.nhs.uk/statistics-and-data-collections/health-and-lifestyles-related-surveys/infant-feeding-survey/infant-feeding-survey-2005.

Bonnar J, Franklin M, Nott P N, McNeilly A S. (1975) Effect of breastfeeding on pituitary – ovarian function after childbirth. *British Medical Journal* **iv**: 82–4.

Borst C G. (1995) *Catching Babies: The professionalization of childbirth 1870–1920*. Cambridge MA; London: Harvard University Press.

Britten J, McInnes R J. (1999) *Promotion and Support for Breastfeeding: 1967– 1999: A summary of action in the UK, Scotland and Glasgow*, PEACH paper no. 8. Glasgow: Department of Child Health.

Broadfoot M, Britten J, Tappin D M, MacKenzie J M. (2005) The Baby-friendly Hospital Initiative and breastfeeding rates in Scotland. *Archives of Disease in Childhood. Fetal and Neonatal Edition* **90**: F114–16.

Buchanan R. (1975) Breastfeeding: aid to infant health and fertility control. *Population Reports Series J: Family Planning Programs* **4**: 49–66.

Cadogan W. (1748) *An Essay Upon Nursing and the Management of Children, From Their Birth to Three Years of Age*. London: J Roberts.

Campbell H, Jones I G. (1994) *Breastfeeding in Scotland*. Glasgow: Scottish Needs Assessment Programme, Scottish Forum for Public Health Medicine.

Campbell H, Jones I G. (1996) Promoting breastfeeding: a view of the current position and a proposed agenda for action in Scotland. *Journal of Public Health Medicine* **18**: 406–14.

Cattaneo A, Buzzetti R. (2001) Effect on rates of breastfeeding of training for the Baby-friendly Hospital Initiative. *British Medical Journal.* **323**: 1358–62.

Cautley E. (1896) *The Natural and Artificial Methods of Feeding Infants and Young Children*. London: Churchill.

Chalmers I, Enkin M, Keirse M J N C. (eds) (1989) *Effective Care in Pregnancy and Childbirth*, Vol. 1: *Pregnancy*; Vol. 2: *Childbirth*. Oxford: Oxford University Press.

Chambers T L. (1999) John David Baum. *Munk's Roll*. Heritage Centre, www. rcplondon.ac.uk/heritage/munksroll/munk_details.asp?ID=4965 (visited 17 June 2008).

Cheadle W B. (1889) *On the Principles and Exact Conditions to be Observed in the Artificial Feeding of Infants*. London: Smith Elder.

Chetley A. (1979) *The Baby Killer Scandal: A War on Want investigation into the promotion and sale of powdered baby milks in the third world*. London: War on Want.

Christie D A, Tansey E M. (eds) (2001a) Origins of Neonatal Intensive Care. *Wellcome Witnesses to Twentieth Century Medicine,* vol. 9. London: The Wellcome Trust Centre for the History of Medicine at UCL. Freely available online at www.ucl.ac.uk/histmed/publications/wellcome-witnesses/index. html or following the links to Publications/Wellcome Witnesses from www. ucl.ac.uk/histmed.

Christie D A, Tansey E M. (eds) (2001b) Maternal Care. *Wellcome Witnesses to Twentieth Century Medicine,* vol. 12. London: The Wellcome Trust Centre for the History of Medicine at UCL. Freely available online at www.ucl. ac.uk/histmed/publications/wellcome-witnesses/index.html or following the links to Publications/Wellcome Witnesses from www.ucl.ac.uk/histmed.

Christie D A, Tansey E M. (eds) (2003) Genetic testing. *Wellcome Witnesses to Twentieth Century Medicine,* vol. 17. London: Wellcome Trust Centre for the History of Medicine at UCL. Freely available online at www.ucl.ac.uk/ histmed/publications/wellcome-witnesses/index.html or following the links to Publications/Wellcome Witnesses from www.ucl.ac.uk/histmed.

Church R C, Tansey E M. (2007) *Burroughs Wellcome and Co.: Knowledge, trust, profit and the transformation of the British pharmaceutical industry, 1880– 1940.* Lancaster: Crucible Books.

Claeson M, Waldman R J. (2000) The evolution of child health programmes in developing countries: From targeting diseases to targeting people. *Bulletin of the World Health Organization* **78**: 1234–45.

Clark C. (1996) *Unicef for Beginners.* New York NY: Writers and Readers Publishing, Inc.

Cockburn F, Brown J K, Belton N R, Forfar J O. (1973) Neonatal convulsions associated with primary disturbance of calcium, phosphorus, and magnesium metabolism. *Archives of Disease in Childhood* **48**: 99–108.

Coovadia H M, Rollins N C, Bland R M, Little K, Coutsoudis A, Bennish M L, Newell M L. (2007) Mother-to-child transmission of HIV-1 infection during exclusive breastfeeding in the first six months of life: An intervention cohort study. *Lancet* **369**: 1107–16.

Cow and Gate (1989) *Ten Years of Infant Feeding, 1974–84.* Trowbridge, Wilts: Cow and Gate Medical Department.

Coward W A, Paul A A, Prentice A M. (1984) The impact of malnutrition on human lactation: observations from community studies. *Federation Proceedings* **43**: 2432–7.

Coward W A, Sawyer M B, Whitehead R C, Prentice A M, Evans J. (1979) New method for measuring milk intakes in breastfed babies. *Lancet* **ii**: 13–14.

Cowie A T. (1999) *The Development of Dairy Science at the National Institute for Research in Dairying.* Cambridge: Cambridge University Press.

Cowie A T, Tindal J S. (1971) *The Physiology of Lactation.* London: Edward Arnold.

Cowie A T, Forsyth I A, Hart I C. (1980) *Hormonal Control of Lactation.* Berlin: Springer-Verlag.

Cox J W. (1978) Effect of supplementary feeding on infant growth in an Aboriginal family. *Journal of Biosocial Science* **10**: 429–36.

Crossland D S, Richmond S, Hudson M, Smith K, Abu-Harb M. (2008) Weight change in the term baby in the first two weeks of life. *Acta Paediatrica* **97**: 425–9.

Dally A. (1968) *Cicely: The story of a doctor.* London: Gollancz.

Daly S E J, Kent J C, Huynh D Q, Owens R A, Alexander B F, Ng K C, Hartmann P E. (1992) The determination of short-term breast volume changes and the rate of synthesis of human milk using computerized breast measurement. *Experimental Physiology* **77**: 79–87.

Davies P A, Robinson R J, Scopes J W, Tizard J P M, Wigglesworth J S. (1972) Medical Care of Newborn Babies. Clinics in Developmental Medicine Series No. 44. London: Heinemann (for) Spastics International Medical Publications.

Department of Health (DoH). (1970) *Recommended Dietary Allowances.* London: DoH.

DoH. (2002) *Infant Feeding 2000: A summary report.* London: Department of Health. Freely available at www.dh.gov.uk/en/Publicationsandstatistics/Publications/PublicationsPolicyAndGuidance/DH_4008114 (visited 16 June 2008).

DoH, Committee on Medical Aspects of Food Policy (COMA). (1994) *Weaning and the Weaning Diet: Report of the Working Group on the weaning diet.* Report on health and social subjects, no. 45. London: HMSO.

DoH, Scottish Office. (1996) *UK Baby Friendly Initiative,* 12 July 1996. Circular SODH/CNO/(96)7.

DoH/UNICEF UK Baby Friendly Initiative. (1993) *Memorandum of Understanding between the National Breastfeeding Working Group and the UNICEF UK Baby Friendly Initiative.* London: Department of Health/ UNICEF UK Baby Friendly Initiative

Department of Health and Social Security (DHSS). (1980) *Present Day Practice in Infant Feeding: 1980. Report of a working party of the Panel on Child Nutrition Committee on Medical Aspects of Food Policy,* Second report. DHSS Report on Health and Social Subjects no. 20. London: HMSO.

DHSS. (1988) *Present Day Practice in Infant Feeding: 1988. Report of a Working Party of the Panel on Child Nutrition Committee on Medical Aspects of Food Policy,* Third report. DHSS Report on Health and Social Subjects no. 32. London: HMSO.

DHSS. (2004) *Breastfeeding Strategy for Northern Ireland.* Belfast: DHSS.

DHSS, Committee on Medical Aspects of Food Policy (COMA). (1977) *The Composition of Mature Human Milk: Report of a Working Party of the Committee on Medical Aspects of Food Policy,* DHSS Report on Health and Social Subjects no. 12. London: HMSO.

DHSS, COMA, Working Party on the Composition of Foods for Infants and Young Children. (1980) *Artificial Feeds for the Young Infant. Report of the Working Party.* Report on Health and Social Subjects no. 18. London: HMSO.

Dewey K G, Peerson J M, Brown K H, Krebs N F, Michaelsen K F, Persson L A, Salmenpera L, Whitehead R G, Yeung D L. (1995) Growth of breastfed infants deviates from current reference data: A pooled analysis of US, Canadian, and European data sets. World Health Organization Working Group on Infant Growth. *Pediatrics* **96**: 495–503.

Dick-Read G. (1942) *Revelation of Childbirth: The principles and practice of natural childbirth.* London: Heinemann Medical Books. US editions (1944–) and later British editions (1951–) have the title: *Childbirth Without Fear.*

Dick-Read G. (2004) *Childbirth Without Fear: The principles and practice of natural childbirth.* London: Pinter & Martin. Original and unabridged edn.

Dingwall-Fordyce A. (1908) *Diet in Infancy.* London: William Green.

Dwork D. (1987a) The milk option: An aspect of the history of the infant welfare movement in England 1898–1908. *Medical History* **31**: 51–69.

Dwork D (1987b) *War is Good for Babies and Other Young Children: A history of the infant and child welfare movement in England 1898–1918.* London: Tavistock Publications.

Dykes F. (2006) *Breastfeeding in Hospital: Mothers, midwives and the production line.* London: Routledge.

Edmond K M, Zandoh C, Quigley M A, Amenga-Etego S, Owusu-Agyei S, Kirkwood B R. (2006) Delayed Breastfeeding initiation increases risk of neonatal mortality. *Pediatrics* **117**: e380–6.

Erlichman J. (1990) Don't speak out, nutrition experts told. *Guardian* (September 11).

Family Health International. (1988) Consensus statement: breastfeeding as a family planning method. *Lancet* **332**: 1204–5.

Farquharson J, Cockburn F, Patrick W A, Jamieson E C, Logan R W. (1992) Infant cerebral cortex phospholipid fatty-acid composition and diet. *Lancet* **340**: 810–1.

Farquharson J, Jamieson E C, Abbasi K A, Patrick W J, Logan R W, Cockburn F. (1995) Effect of diet on the fatty acid composition of the major phospholipids of infant cerebral cortex. *Archives of Disease in Childhood* **72**: 198–203.

Ferguson A E, Tappin D M, Girdwood R W, Kennedy R, Cockburn F. (1994) Breastfeeding in Scotland. *British Medical Journal* **308**: 824–5.

Ferguson A H, Weaver L T, Nicolson M. (2006) The Glasgow Corporation milk depot 1904–1910 and its role in infant welfare: an end or a means? *Social History of Medicine* **19**: 443–60.

Fildes V. (1985) *Breasts, Bottles and Babies: A history of infant feeding.* Edinburgh: Edinburgh University Press.

Fildes V. (1988) *Wet Nursing: A history from antiquity to the present.* Oxford: Basil Blackwell Ltd.

Fildes V. (1998) Infant feeding practices and infant mortality in England, 1900–19. *Continuity and Change* **13**: 251–80.

Finger W R. (1996) Research confirms LAM's effectiveness: contraceptive update. *Network* **17**: 12–14, 24.

Fisher C. (1985) The puerperium and breastfeeding. In Marsh G N. (ed.) *Modern Obstetrics in General Practice.* Oxford: Oxford University Press, 325–48.

Forsyth D. (1911) The history of infant-feeding from Elizabethan times. *Proceedings of the Royal Society for History of Medicine* **4**: 110–41.

Forsyth I A. (1970) The detection of lactogenic activity in human blood by bioassay. *Journal of Endocrinology* **46**: iv–v.

Forsyth I A. (2003) In memoriam: Alfred T Cowie (1916–2003). *Journal of Mammary Gland Biology and Neoplasia* **8**: 487–9.

Gallivan S. (2000) *Report to the Bristol Royal Infirmary Inquiry: Key directions for the future in monitoring clinical performance: A discussion paper.* November 2000. UCL, Clinical Operational Research Unit, Department of Mathematics, Paper no. 579, funded by the Bristol Royal Infirmary Inquiry.

Granshaw L, Porter R. (1989) *The Hospital in History.* London; New York, NY: Routledge.

Gunther M H D. (1953) Sore nipples. *Medical World* **79**: 571–5.

Gunther M H D. (1963) The comparative merits of breast- and bottle-feeding. *Proceedings of the Nutrition Society* **22**: 134–9.

Gunther M H D. (1970) *Infant Feeding.* London: Methuen. Revised edn, Penguin, 1973.

Gunther M H D. (1975) The neonate's immunity gap, breastfeeding and cot death. *Lancet* **i**: 441–2.

Guthrie R. (1996) The introduction of newborn screening for phenylketonuria: a personal history. *European Journal of Pediatrics.* **155** (Suppl.): S4–5.

Hanson L Å. (2004) *Immunobiology of Human Milk: How breastfeeding protects babies.* Amarillo, TX: Pharmasoft Publishing.

Heinig M J. (1998) The 'Bellagio Consensus': ten years later. *Journal of Human Lactation* **14**: 185–6.

Helsing E, Häggkvist A-P. (forthcoming) *Understanding Breastfeeding.*

Helsing E, Savage F. (1982) *Breastfeeding in Practice: A manual for healthworkers.* Oxford; New York, NY: Oxford University Press.

Hofvander Y. (2005) Breastfeeding and the Baby-friendly Hospital Initiative (BFHI): Organization, response and outcome in Sweden and other countries. *Acta Paediatrica* **94**: 1012–16.

Holt L E. (1901) *The Care and Feeding of Children.* New York, NY: Appleton.

Holt L E. (1957) *The Good Housekeeping Book of Baby and Child Care.* New York, NY: Popular Library, Inc.

Hopkins D, Emmett P, Steer C, Rogers I, Noble S, Emond A. (2007) Infant feeding in the second six months of life related to iron status: an observational study. *Archives of Disease in Childhood* **92**: 850–4.

Howie P W, Forsyth J S, Ogston S A, Clark A, Florey C D. (1990) Protective effect of breastfeeding against infection. *British Medical Journal* **300**: 11–16.

Howie P W, McNeilly A S, Houston M J, Cook A, Boyle H. (1981) Effect of supplementary food on suckling patterns and ovarian activity during lactation. *British Medical Journal* **283**: 757–9.

Hytten F E. (1954) Clinical and chemical studies in human lactation. VII. The effect of differences in yield and composition of milk on the infant's weight gain and the duration of breastfeeding. *British Medical Journal* **i**: 1410–13.

Illingworth R S, Stone D G, Jowett G H, Scott J F. (1952) Self-demand feeding in a maternity unit. *Lancet* **i**: 683–7.

Iyer N P, Srinivasan R, Evans K, Ward L, Cheung W Y, Matthes J W. (2007) Impact of early weighing policy on neonatal hypernatraemic dehydration and breastfeeding. *Archives of Disease in Childhood* **93**: 797–9.

Janas L M, Picciano M F, Hatch T F. (1998) Indices of protein metabolism in term infants fed human milk, whey-predominant formula, or cows'-milk formula. *Pediatrics* **75**: 775–84.

Jelliffe D B, Jelliffe E F P. (1978) *Human Milk in the Modern World: Psychosocial, nutritional and economic significance.* Oxford: Oxford University Press.

Jelliffe D B, Jelliffe E F P. (1979) Adequacy of breastfeeding. *Lancet* **ii**: 691–2.

Jensen R G, Neville M. (eds). (1985) *Human Lactation: Milk components and methodologies.* New York, NY: Plenum Press.

Jones G, Steketee R W, Black R E, Bhutta Z A, Morris S S. Bellagio Child Survival Study Group. (2003) How many child deaths can we prevent this year? *Lancet* **362**: 65–71.

Kennedy K I, Rivera R, McNeilly A S. (1989) Consensus statement on the use of breastfeeding as a family planning method. *Contraception* **39**: 477–96.

King J, Ashworth A. (1987a) *Changes in Infant Feeding Practices in Malaysia.* Occasional paper no. 7. London: London School of Hygiene and Tropical Medicine.

King J, Ashworth A. (1987b) *Changes in Infant Feeding Practices in the Caribbean.* Occasional paper no. 8. London: London School of Hygiene and Tropical Medicine.

King J, Ashworth A. (1987c) *Changes in Infant Feeding Practices in Nigeria.* Occasional paper no. 9. London: London School of Hygiene and Tropical Medicine.

Kippley S. (1973) *Breastfeeding and Natural Child Spacing: The ecology of natural mothering.* New York, NY: Harper & Row.

Kitzinger S. (1962) *The Experience of Childbirth.* London: Gollancz.

Kitzinger S. (1980) *The Experience of Breastfeeding.* London: Penguin.

Kramer M S, Chalmers B, Hodnett E D, Sevkovskaya Z, Dzikovich I, Shapiro S, Collet J P, Vanilovich I, Mezen I, Ducruet T, Shishko G, Zubovich V, Mknuik D, Gluchanina E, Dombrovskiy V, Ustinovitch A, Kot T, Bogdanovich N, Ovchinikova L, Helsing E. (2001) Promotion of Breastfeeding Intervention Trial (PROBIT). A randomized trial in the Republic of Belarus. *Journal of the American Medical Association* **285**: 413–20.

La Leche League International. (1963) *The Womanly Art of Breastfeeding.* Franklin Park, IL: La Leche International.

La Leche League International. (2004) *The Womanly Art of Breastfeeding*. 7th revised edn. London: Penguin.

Labbok M H, Hight-Laukaran V, Peterson A E, Fletcher V, Von Hertzen H, Van Look P F. (1997) Multicenter Study of the lactational amenorrhea method (LAM): I. Efficacy, duration, and implications for clinical application. *Contraception* **55**: 327–36.

Ladd-Taylor M. (1986) *Raising a Baby the Government Way: Mothers' letters to the Children's Bureau, 1915–1932*. New Brunswick, NJ: Rutgers University Press.

Laing I A, Wong C M. (2002) Hypernatraemia in the first few days: Is the incidence rising? *Archives of Disease in Childhood* Fetal and Neonatal edn **87**: F158–62.

Lande B. (2003) *Spedkost 6 Måneder. Landsomfattende Kostholdsundersøkelse Blant Spedbarn i Norge*. Oslo: Sosial-og helsedirektoratet.

Latham M. (2007) Obituary and personal remembrances: Patrice Jelliffe, died 14 March 2007. *SCN News* **35**: 72–3.

Laurence B M. (1994) Derrick Brian Jelliffe. *Munk's Roll* **9**: 271–3.

Liestøl K, Rosenberg M, Walløe L. (1988) Breastfeeding practice in Norway 1860–1984. *Journal of Biosocial Science* **20**: 45–58.

Lincoln D W, Paisley A C. (1982) Neuroendocrine control of milk ejection. *Journal of Reproduction and Fertility* **65**: 571–86.

Linzell J L. (1972) Milk yield, energy loss in milk, and mammary gland weight in different species. *Dairy Science Abstracts* **34**: 351–60.

Macy E, Kelly H J, Sloan R F. (1953) *The Composition of Milk*, Publication 254, Washington, DC: National Academy of Science.

MAIN Trial Collaborative Group. (1994) Preparing for breastfeeding: treatment of inverted and non-protractile nipples in preganacy. *Midwifery* **10**: 200–14.

Martin J. (1978) *Infant Feeding 1975: Attitudes and practice in England and Wales*. London: HMSO.

Martin J, Monk J. (1982) *Infant Feeding: 1980: A survey carried out for the DHSS by the OPCS*. London: HMSO.

Mayes M. (1937) *Handbook for Midwives,* 1st edn. London: Baillière, Tindall & Cox.

McCleary G F. (1933) *The Early History of the Infant Welfare Movement.* London: Lewis and Company.

McNeilly A S, McNeilly J R. (1978) Spontaneous milk ejection during lactation and its possible relevance to success of breastfeeding. *British Medical Journal* **ii**: 466–8.

McNeilly A S, Robinson I C, Houston M J, Howie P W. (1983) Release of oxytocin and prolactin in response to suckling. *British Medical Journal* **286**: 257–9.

Meckel R A. (1990) *Save the Babies: American public health reform and the prevention of infant mortality 1850–1929.* Baltimore, MD; London: Johns Hopkins University Press.

Mepham T B. (1993) Humanizing milk: the formulation of artificial feeds for infants (1850–1910). *Medical History* **37**: 225–49.

Michaelsen K F, Weaver L, Branca F, Robertson A. (eds) (2003) *Feeding and Nutrition of Infants and Young Children: Guidelines for the WHO European region, with emphasis on the former Soviet countries.* Copenhagen: World Health Organization. Freely available at www.euro.who.int/InformationSources/Publications/Catalogue/20010914_21 (visited 8 June 2008).

Minchin M K. (1989) *Breastfeeding Matters: What we need to know about infant feeding.* Sydney: Allen & Unwin; Armadale, Victoria, Australia: Alma Publications.

Morton J. (1989) The clinical usefulness of breast-milk sodium in the assessment of lactogenesis. *Pediatrics* **93**: 802–6.

The National Assembly for Wales. (2001) *Investing in a Better Start: Promoting breastfeeding in Wales.* Cardiff: National Assembly for Wales.

National Breastfeeding Working Group. (1995) *Breastfeeding: Good practice guidance to the NHS.* London: Department of Health.

National Childbirth Trust (NCT), United Nations Children's Fund (UNICEF UK). (2005) *Legal Loophole Allows Banned Formula Advertising to Mothers.* Research paper, 19 September 2005. Freely available at www.babyfriendly.org.uk/items/item_detail.asp?item=47 (visited 11 August 2008).

National Institute for health and Clinical Excellence (NICE). (2008) *Improving the Nutrition of Pregnant and Breastfeeding Mothers and Children in Low Income Households.* London: NICE. See www.nice.org.uk/nicemedia/pdf/PH011guidance.pdf (visited 18 February 2009).

Nestlè. (c.1950) *Nestlè in Profile.* Switzerland: Nestlè.

Newman G. (1906) *Infant Mortality.* London: Methuen.

Oddie S, Richmond S, Couthard M. (2001) Hypernatraemic dehydration and breastfeeding: a population study. *Archives of Disease in Childhood* **87**: 318–20.

Oppé T E. (1961) *Modern Textbook of Paediatrics for Nurses.* London: Heinemann.

Oppé T E, Arneil C C, Creary R D G, Lloyd J K, Stroud C E, Wharton B A, Widdowson E M, Department of Health and Social Security, Committee on Medical Aspects of Food Policy. (1974) *Present-day Practice in Infant Feeding.* DHSS Report on Health and Social Subjects no. 9. London: HMSO.

Peaker M, Linzell J L. (1975) Citrate in milk: a harbinger of lactogenesis. *Nature* **253**: 464.

Plewis I. (2004) *Millennium Cohort Study: Technical report on sampling.* London: Institute of Education, University of London. UK Data Archive, UK Millennium Cohort Study: First Survey, 2001–2003 (SN 4683).

Pontifical Academy of Science, Working Group. (1994) Breastfeeding: science and society, 11–13 May 1994, Summary Report. *Scripta Varia* **28**: 35. Available at www.vatican.va/roman_curia/pontifical_academies/acdscien/own/documents/rc_acdsci_doc_190999_publications_it.html (visited 18 June 2008).

Pontifical Academy of Science, Working Group. (1995) Breastfeeding: Science and society. 11–13 May 1995, *Scripta Varia* **94**: iv–453. Available at www.vatican.va/roman_curia/pontifical_academies/acdscien/own/documents/rc_acdsci_doc_190999_publications_it.html (visited 18 June 2008).

Pope John Paul II. (1995) *Address to the Pontifical Academy of Sciences,* 12 May 1995. San Antonio, Italy: The Couple To Couple League For Natural Family Planning. Available at http://cclsanantonio.org/resources/article.asp?cid=1&AID=72 (visited 18 February 2009).

Prentice A M, Whitehead R G, Roberts S B, Paul A A, Watkinson M, Prentice A, Watkinson A A. (1980) Dietary supplementation of Gambian nursing mothers and lactational performance. *Lancet* **ii**: 886–8.

Pritchard E. (1907) *Infant Education.* London: Marylebone Health Society.

Pritchard E. (1938) *The Infant: A handbook of modern treatment.* London: Edward Arnold.

Quigley M A, Kelly Y J, Sacker A. (2007) Breastfeeding and hospitalization for diarrheal and respiratory infection in the UK Millennium Cohort Study. *Pediatrics* **119**: e837-42.

Renfrew M J, Hall D. (2008) Enabling women to breastfeed is a challenge for the health professionals. *British Medical Journal* **337**: 1066–7.

Renfrew M J, McCandlish R M. (1992) With women: new steps in research in midwifery. In Roberts H. (ed.) (1992) *Women's Health Matters.* London: Routledge: 81–98.

Renfrew M J, Fisher C, Arms S. (2004) *Bestfeeding: How to breastfeed your baby,* 3rd edn. Berkeley, CA: Ten Speed Press.

Reynolds L A, Tansey E M. (eds) (2005) Prenatal corticosteroids for reducing morbidity and mortality after preterm birth. *Wellcome Witnesses to Twentieth Century Medicine,* vol. 25. London: Wellcome Trust Centre for the History of Medicine at UCL. Freely available online at www.ucl.ac.uk/histmed/ publications/wellcome-witnesses/index.html or following the links to Publications/Wellcome Witnesses from www.ucl.ac.uk/histmed

Richmond S. (2003) Hypernatraemic dehydration: excess sodium is not the cause. [Letter] *Archives of Disease in Childhood* **88**: F349–50.

Ronchi F P, Góngora Y, Lopez J. (1976) Evaluation of supplementary feeding programmes assisted by the World Food Programme. *Food and Nutrition* **2**: 19–25.

Rosenberg M. (1989) Breastfeeding and infant mortality in Norway 1860–1930. *Journal of Biosocial Science* **21**: 335–48.

Rosenberg M. (1991) *On the Relation Between Living Conditions and Variables Linked to Reproduction in Norway, 1860–1984.* Oslo: PhD thesis, University of Oslo, Department of Informatic [doktoravhandling].

Rotch T M. (1983) The general principles underlying all good methods of infant feeding. *Boston Medical and Surgical Journal* **129**: 505.

Routh C H F. (1879) *Infant Feeding and its Influence on Life*, 3rd edn. London: John Churchill.

Rowland M G. (1986) The weanling's dilemma: are we making progress? *Acta Paediatrica Scandanavia* **323** (Suppl.): 33–42.

Rowland M G, Paul A A, Whitehead R G. (1981) Lactation and infant nutrition. *British Medical Bulletin* **37**: 77–82.

Royal College of Midwives, Breastfeeding Working Group (Inch S, Fisher C, Garforth S, Salariya E, Woolridge M with contributions by Rowe J, Kerr M). (1988) *Successful Breastfeeding*. London: Royal College of Midwives. Second edn, 1993; third edn, 2002.

Sachs M, Dykes F, Carter B. (2005) Weight monitoring of breastfed babies in the UK: centile charts, scales and weighing frequency. *Maternal and Child Nutrition* **1**: 63–76.

Sachs M Y. (ed.) (1975) *The PAG Compendium. The collected papers issued by the Protein-Calorie Advisory Group of the United Nations System, 1956–73.* Volumes C1 & C2 (Food science and technology, specific). New York, NY: Worldmark Press/John Wiley & Sons.

Sadler S H. (1909) *Infant Feeding by Artificial Means: A scientific and practical treatise on the dietetics of infancy.* London: Routledge.

Salariya E M, Easton P M, Cater J I. (1978) Duration of breastfeeding after early initiation and frequent feeding. *Lancet* **ii**: 1141–3.

Savage W. (1986) *A Savage Enquiry.* London: Virago Press Ltd.

Savage W. (2007) *Birth and Power: A Savage enquiry revisited. An examination of who controls childbirth and who controls doctors.* Middlesex University Press.

Scrimshaw N S, Taylor C E, Gordon J E. (1968) *Interaction of Nutrition and Infection,* WHO Monograph no. 57. Geneva: WHO.

Short R V. (1976) Lactation: the central control of reproduction. *Ciba Clinical Symposia* (**45**): 73–86.

Short R V. (1992) Breastfeeding, fertility and population growth. In United Nations administrative committee on coordination, subcommittee on nutrition. *Nutrition and Population Links: Breastfeeding, family planning and child health.* Papers from the ACC/SCN 18th Session Symposium, (ACC/SCN Symposium Report, Nutrition Policy Discussion Paper no. 11). Geneva: United Nations: 33–46.

Short R V, Lewis P R, Renfrew M B, Shaw G. (1991) Contraceptive effects of extended lactational amenorrhea: beyond the Bellagio Consensus. *Lancet* **337**: 715–7.

Sloper K, Baum D. (1974) Proceedings: patterns of infant feeding in Oxford. *Archives of Disease in Childhood* **49**: 749.

Smale M. (2004) *Training Breastfeeding Supporters: An enabling approach.* Sheffield: WICH Research Group.

Smith K, Joshi H. (2002) The Millennium Cohort Study. *Population Trends* **117**: 30–4.

Stanway P, Stanway A. (1978) *Breast is Best: A common sense approach to breastfeeding.* London: Pan Books.

Stoppard M. (1982) *A Complete Guide to Baby Care.* London: Octopus Ltd.

Symonds C, Burningham S. (1989) *Ten Years of Infant Feeding, 1974–84.* Trowbridge, Wilts: Cow and Gate Medical Department.

Tanner J M, Whitehouse R H. (1973) Height and weight charts from birth to 5 years allowing for length of gestation. *Archives of Disease in Childhood:* **48**: 786–9.

Tanner J M, Whitehouse R H, Takaishi M. (1966a) Standards from birth to maturity for height, weight, height velocity and weight velocity: British children, 1965. I. *Archives of Disease in Childhood* **41**: 454–71.

Tanner J M, Whitehouse R H, Takaishi M. (1966b) Standards from birth to maturity for height, weight, height velocity and weight velocity: British children, 1965. II. *Archives of Disease in Childhood* **41**: 613–35.

Tansey E M, Christie D A. (eds) (2000) Looking at the Unborn: Historical aspects of obstetric ultrasound. *Wellcome Witnesses to Twentieth Century Medicine*, vol. 5. London: The Wellcome Trust. Freely available online at www.ucl.ac.uk/histmed/publications/wellcome-witnesses/index.html or following the links to Publications/Wellcome Witnesses from www.ucl.ac.uk/histmed.

Tappin D M, Girdwood R W, Follett E A, Kennedy R, Brown A J, Cockburn F. (1991) Prevalence of maternal HIV infection in Scotland based on unlinked anonymous testing of newborn babies. *Lancet* **337**: 1565–7.

Tappin D M, Girdwood R W, Follett E A, Kennedy R, Brown A J, Cockburn F. (1993) Prevalence of maternal HIV infection in Scotland based on unlinked anonymous testing of newborn babies: Update. *Scottish Medical Journal* **38**: 16–17.

Thomson A M, Hytten F E, Billewicz W Z. (1970) The energy cost of human lactation. *British Journal of Nutrition* **24**: 565–72.

Trowell H C, Jelliffe D B. (1958) *Diseases of Children in the Subtropics and Tropics*. London: Edward Arnold.

Truby King F. (1913) *Feeding and Care of Baby*. Sydney: Whitcombe and Tombs, London: Macmillan.

UNICEF, UK Baby Friendly Initiative (1999) *Towards National, Regional and Local Strategies for Breastfeeding*. Freely available at www.babyfriendly.org.uk/pdfs/strategy.pdf (visited 18 June 2008).

United Nations. (1996) *Food and Nutrition Bulletin* **17**. Tokyo, Japan: United Nations University. Freely available at www.unu.edu/unupress/food/8f174e/8F174E00.htm#Contents (visited 11 August 2008).

Vallena C, Savage F. (1998) *Evidence for the Ten Steps to Successful Breastfeeding*. Geneva: WHO.

Vincent R. (1910) *The Nutrition of the Infant*, 3rd edn. London: Baillière, Tindall and Cox.

Wahlqvist M. (ed.) (1995) *Proceedings of the XV International Congress of Nutrition, Adelaide, September 1993*. Adelaide: IUNS.

Wake Y. (2006) *Compliance with the International Code of Marketing of Breast-milk Substitutes in Parenting Magazines in the UK*. MSc Project. The London School of Hygiene and Tropical Medicine.

Wakerley J B, Lincoln D W. (1971) Intermittent release of oxytocin during suckling in the rat. *Nature New Biology* **233**: 180–1.

Walker-Smith J A. (1997) Children in hospital. In Loudon I (ed.) *Western Medicine: An illustrated history.* Oxford; New York, NY: Oxford University Press.

Waller H K. (1952) The importance of breastfeeding. *British Journal of Nutrition* **6**: 10–15.

Waterlow J C, Thomson A M. (1979) Observations on the adequacy of breastfeeding. *Lancet* **ii**: 238–42.

Waterlow J C, Ashworth A, Griffiths M. (1980) Faltering in infant growth in less-developed countries. *Lancet* **ii**: 1176–8.

Weaver L T. (2006) The emergence of our modern understanding of infant nutrition and feeding 1750–1900. *Current Paediatrics* **16**: 342–7.

Weaver L T. (2008) Infant welfare, philanthropy and entrepreneurship in Glasgow: Sister Laura's Infant Food Company. *Journal of the Royal College of Physicians of Edinburgh* **38**: 179–86.

West C P, McNeilly A S. (1979) Hormonal profiles in lactating and non-lactating women immediately after delivery and their relationship to breast engorgement. *British Journal of Obstetrics and Gynaecology* **86**: 501–6.

Whitehead R G. (1969) Factors which may affect the biochemical response to protein–calorie malnutrition. In Mural A V. (ed.) *Protein–Calorie Malnutrition.* Berlin: Springer: 38–47.

Whitehead R G. (1985) Infant physiology, nutritional requirements and lactational adequacy. *American Journal of Clinical Nutrition* **41**: 447–458.

Whitehead R G, Paul A A. (1984) Growth charts and the assessment of infant feeding practices in the western world and in developing countries. *Early Human Development* **9**: 187–207.

Whitehead R G, Prentice A. (eds) (1991) *New Techniques in Nutrition Research.* San Diego, CA: Academic Press.

Whitehead R G, Paul A A, Cole T J. (1981) A critical analysis of measured food energy intakes during infancy and early childhood in comparison with current international recommendations. *Journal of Human Nutrition* **35**: 339–48.

Whitehead R G, Rowland M G, Hutton M, Prentice A M, Müller E, Paul A. (1978) Factors influencing lactation performance in rural Gambian mothers. *Lancet* **ii**: 178–81.

Wickes I G. (1953) A history of infant feeding: Part 1. *Archives of Disease in Childhood* **28**: 151–8.

Williams C D. (1933) A nutritional disease of childhood associated with a maize diet. *Archives of Disease in Childhood* **8**: 423–33.

Williams C D. (1935) Kwashiorkor: A nutritional disease of children associated with a maize diet. *Lancet* **ii**: 1151–2.

Williams C D, Jelliffe D B. (1972) *Mother and Child Health: Delivering the services*. London, New York, NY: Oxford University Press.

Willox J, Barr W. (2004) *Ian Donald – A Memoir*. London: RCOG Press.

World Health Organization (WHO). (1974) *Twenty-seventh World Health Assembly, Resolution WHA27.43*. Geneva: WHO.

WHO. (1978) *Thirty-first World Health Assembly, Resolution WHA31.47*. Geneva: WHO.

WHO. (1981a) *Contemporary Patterns of Breastfeeding*. Report on the WHO Collaborative Study on Breastfeeding. Geneva: WHO.

WHO. (1981b) *The International Code of Marketing of Breast-milk Substitutes*. Geneva: WHO. Freely available at www.ibfan.org/site2005/Pages/article.php?art_id=52&iui=1 (visited 27 January 2009).

WHO. (2003) *Global Strategy for Infant and Young Child Feeding*. Geneva: WHO. Freely available at www.who.int/nutrition/topics/global_strategy/en/index.html (visited 18 June 2008).

WHO, Collaborative Study Team. (2000) Effect of breastfeeding on infant mortality due to infectious diseases in less developed countries: A pooled analysis. *Lancet* **355**: 451–5.

WHO. Multicentre Growth Reference Study Group. (2006) WHO child growth standards based on length/height, weight and age. *Acta Paediatrica: Suppl.* **450**: 76–85.

WHO, Task Force on Methods for the Natural Regulation of Fertility. (1998a) The WHO Multinational Study of Breastfeeding and Lactational Amenorrhea. I. Description of infant feeding patterns and of the return of menses. *Fertility and Sterility* **70**: 448–60.

WHO, Task Force on Methods for the Natural Regulation of Fertility. (1998b) The WHO Multinational Study of Breastfeeding and Lactational Amenorrhea. II. Factors associated with the length of amenorrhea. *Fertility and Sterility* **70**: 461–71.

WHO, Task Force on Methods for the Natural Regulation of Fertility. (1999a) The WHO Multinational Study of Breastfeeding and Lactational Amenorrhea. III. Pregnancy during breastfeeding. *Fertility and Sterility* **72**: 431–40.

WHO, Task Force on Methods for the Natural Regulation of Fertility. (1999b) The WHO Multinational Study of Breastfeeding and Lactational Amenorrhea. IV. Postpartum bleeding and lochia in breastfeeding women. *Fertility and Sterility* **72**: 441–7.

WHO/UNICEF. (1989) *Ten Steps to Successful Breastfeeding in Protecting, Promoting and Supporting Breastfeeding: The special role of maternity services. A joint WHO/UNICEF statement.* Geneva: WHO.

Wolf J H. (2001) *Don't Kill Your Baby: Public health and the decline of breastfeeding in the nineteenth and twentieth centuries.* Columbus, OH: Ohio State University Press.

Woolridge M W. (1986) The 'anatomy' of infant sucking. *Midwifery.* **2**: 164–71.

Woolridge M W. (1994) The Baby Friendly Hospital Initiative UK. *Modern Midwife* **4**: 32–3.

Woolridge M W, Ingram J. (2007) Response to a research study on feeding time at the breast. *MIDIRS Midwifery Digest* **17**: 247–51.

Biographical notes*

Mr James Akre

(b. 1944) began his health-and-development career working with rural populations in Turkey and Cameroon (1966–71). After obtaining an MSc in economic and social development (University of Pittsburgh, 1972), he continued his international focus in three UN agencies, including the WHO where he has served for 25 years as technical officer in the department of nutrition. In this capacity he participated in drafting and promoting the adoption of the *International Code of Marketing of Breast-milk Substitutes* (1981); the joint WHO/UNICEF statement on breastfeeding and the special role of maternity services (1989), the foundation for the Baby-friendly Hospital Initiative; and the *Global Strategy for Infant and Young Child Feeding* (2003). Upon retirement in 2004 he was elected to the board of directors of the International Board of Lactation Consultant Examiners (IBLCE).

Professor Elizabeth (Beth) Alder

PhD FBPsS (b. 1944) graduated in psychology at the University of Aberdeen in 1967 and gained a doctorate at the University of Edinburgh in 1971. She worked part-time at the MRC reproductive biology unit, Edinburgh (1975–87) and subsequently held academic posts at Queen Margaret College (1987–95) and Dundee University Medical School (1995–2000) before becoming professor and director of research in the faculty of health sciences at Napier University, Edinburgh. She was president of the International Society of Psychosomatic Obstetrics and Gynaecology (2004–07) and chaired the NHS Health Scotland's breastfeeding expert group in 2006.

Professor Rima D Apple

(b. 1944) received her PhD from the University of Wisconsin-Madison. She was lecturer, State University of New York at Stony Brook (1981–83); member, women's studies program (1983–92) and fellow, department of the history of medicine (1985–92), at the University of Wisconsin-Madison. She subsequently held joint appointments at the University of Wisconsin-Madison school of human ecology, as professor of consumer science (1992–2007); interdisciplinary

---

* Contributors are asked to supply details; other entries are compiled from conventional biographical sources.

studies in human ecology (1996–2007); women's studies (1983–2007) and science and technology (2001–07); and has been an affiliate of the department of the medical history and bioethics since 1992. She was researcher, Wellcome Trust Centre for the History of Medicine at UCL (2004–08); and co-editor of *Advancing the Consumer Interest* (1994–98). and was the ACOG-Ortho fellow in the history of American obstetrics and gynaecology, American College of Obstetricians and Gynaecologists (1996). See Apple (1997, 2006).

Professor John David Baum
FRCP FRCPCH FRCPE
(1940–99) qualified and trained at the university of Birmingham and joined the Hammersmith Hospital, London, as senior house officer and then research fellow, working for Peter Tizard, who was then developing the specialty of neonatal medicine. He moved to the University of Oxford's department of paediatrics where Tizard become chair in 1972 and became interested in nutrition and maternal breast-milks, working with medical physicists and bioengineers in the development of instruments to measure breast-milk flow during feeding. In 1985 he was appointed to the chair of child health at the University of Bristol until his sudden death on a sponsored bike ride to raise money to help children in the Balkans. He was president of the Royal College of Paediatrics and Child Health (1997–99). See Chambers (1999).

Mrs Phyll Buchanan
(b. 1957) trained as a nurse and midwife in the 1970s and worked as a sister in intensive care at Guy's Hospital (1982–84). She has worked in the voluntary sector supporting breastfeeding women for nearly two decades. She was a founder member and trustee of the NCT Breastfeeding Network. As a tutor she has trained and supervised peer supporters in various communities in England and Wales. With her colleague Lorna Hartwell, she has recently been seconded to the Department of Health as an infant feeding best practice adviser.

Professor Forrester Cockburn
CBE FRSE FRCPGlas FRCPEd HonFRCPCH HonFRCSEd
(b. 1934) qualified at the University of Edinburgh in 1959 and had general professional and paediatric training in the Royal Infirmary, Simpson Memorial Maternity Pavilion and Royal Hospital for Sick Children, Edinburgh. Thereafter he was Huntingdon-Hartford research fellow in paediatric metabolic disease, University of Boston, Massachusetts; Nuffield senior research fellow

in neonatal and fetal physiology, University of Oxford; Wellcome senior research fellow in neonatal and paediatric research, University of Edinburgh; senior lecturer, University of Edinburgh; and Samson-Gemmell professor, department of child health, Universtiy of Glasgow (1977–96). He has been chairman of Yorkhill NHS Trust panel on child nutrition, DoH (1985–96); the MRC/DoH phenylketonuria/hypothyroid screening committee (1984–94); the ethics committee of the British Paediatric Association (1978–85); and president of the British (1987–90) and European (1996–98) Associations of Perinatal Medicine; and the Scottish Paediatric Society (1993/4).

Dr Alfred T Cowie

PhD DSc FBiol FRCVS (1916–2003), endocrinologist, qualified at the Royal Veterinary College, Edinburgh, moving to Sir Joseph Barcroft's Cambridge laboratory as a research fellow, working for him and D H Barron on the physiology of fetal sheep. Returning to Edinburgh he continued to study the energy metabolism of pregnant sheep and the digestibility of alkali-treated straw. In 1941 he was appointed to the National Institute for Research in Dairying at Shinfield, near Reading, where he worked with S J Folley and G W Scott-Blair on a pregnancy test for cattle, later becoming interested in lactation. During the war, he worked to improve the productivity of dairy herds by inducing lactation in barren cattle. He was a member of the Ministry of Agriculture, Fisheries and Food's veterinary products committee (1970–77) and editor of the *Journal of Endocrinology* (1981–84). See Cowie (1999); Forsyth (2003).

Ms Rosie Dodds

is a graduate in nutrition and dietetics (1980), with an interest in injustice. Following travel and work in India, Egypt and Sudan, she worked in research preventing postoperative thrombosis and the complications of diabetes. The birth of her son in 1988 prompted her to train as a breastfeeding counsellor with the NCT. This led to work in policy research at the NCT and lobbying to improve support for breastfeeding in the UK.

Mrs Jill Dye

IBCLC (b. 1949) graduated in anthropology from the University of California, Berkeley, (1976) and gained a masters in archaeological sciences at the University of Bradford (1978). As the mother of three children she realized that archaeology was not the career for her and moved into the voluntary sector. In 1988 she became a La Leche League leader; served on the council of directors of La Leche League Great Britain (LLLGB) as director of publications; represented LLLGB on the Joint Breastfeeding Initiative executive committee and steering group; represented LLLGB on the national breastfeeding working group and on the national network of breastfeeding coordinators. She is currently representing LLLGB on the UNICEF Baby Friendly Initiative steering group and is a lactation consultant in private practice in the London area.

Professor Fiona Dykes

ADM RM RGN Cert Ed PhD (b. 1960) qualified as a midwife in 1984 in Chatham, Kent. She practised as a midwife in Kent and East Lancashire. She gained an MA in health research in 1998 at Lancaster University and a PhD from the faculty of medicine at University of Sheffield in 2004. She conducted a critical medical anthropological study of institutional practices of breastfeeding mothers in maternity hospitals in north-west England, later published (Dykes, 2006). She is currently director of the maternal and infant nutrition and nurture unit at the University of Central Lancashire, which she founded in 2000; and adjunct professor at the University of Western Sydney; facilitator for the WHO/

UNICEF *Global Strategy for Infant and Young Child Feeding* (2003) and is currently domain editor for *Maternal and Child Nutrition.*

Ms Hilary English

IBCLC is a breastfeeding counsellor with the National Childbirth Trust, and tutored for them (1987–2008). She was a member of the Royal College of Midwives breastfeeding working group (2000–03). She produces promotional material, photographs and graphics, and trains health professionals in private practice.

Miss Chloe Fisher

MBE NNEB RN RM MTD (b. 1932), a midwife for over 50 years, was the clinical specialist in infant feeding at the John Radcliffe Hospital, Oxford (1991–97). In 1996 she was appointed MBE for her services to infant healthcare, and honorary fellow, Oxford Brookes University (1997). Although retired, she is a volunteer at the Oxford breastfeeding clinic; vice-president of the Royal College of Midwives; an adviser to Le Leche League GB; and was a former adviser to the International Lactation Consultants Association. She is an honorary life member of the National Childbirth Trust; and was consultant to UNICEF/WHO in former Yugoslavia, (1992–97). She has lectured on breastfeeding and chaired the Royal College of Midwives, breastfeeding working group (1988), which produced *Successful Breastfeeding*. See Renfrew *et al.* (2004).

Professor Anna Glasier

CBE MD DSc (b. 1950) trained in obstetrics and gynaecology at Edinburgh and Winchester after qualifying from Bristol University. She subspecialized in reproductive medicine and was a clinical scientist at the MRC unit of reproductive biology, Edinburgh (1989–90). She is lead clinician for sexual health in NHS Lothian region and holds honorary professorships at the universities of Edinburgh and London. She chaired the scientific and technical advisory group of the WHO's human reproductive programme (2004–08).

Professor Lars Hanson

MD PhD HonFRCPCH (b. 1934) trained at Institute Pasteur, Paris, (1958) and the Rockefeller Institute, New York, (1962/3), and interned in paediatrics at Göteborg Hospital and the department of paediatrics, Karolinska Institute, Stockholm, Sweden. He has been a specialist in paediatrics since 1969 and in clinical immunology since 1977; head of the department of immunology, Göteborg University (1969–77); head of the department of clinical immunology (1978–2000), and was a consultant in paediatrics, Göteborg Children's Hospital, until 2000. See Hanson (2004).

Dr Elisabet Helsing

DrMedSci (b. 1940) trained in nutrition physiology at the University of Oslo; was responsible for changes in breastfeeding frequency in Norway where she wrote the pamphlet *How You Breastfeed Your Child: Some advice for the early days* in 1968; started a mother-to-mother support association in 1968, and wrote *The Book About Breastfeeding* in 1970. She became responsible for nutrition in the WHO regional office for Europe (1984–96); received the first Grande Covian Award from the Mediterranean Diet Foundation, Barcelona (1996); the Norwegian King's Gold Medal for services to the people (2003); is an honorary member of the Norwegian (1988) and the Swedish (2003) mother-to-mother breastfeeding support organization; president of the 8th European Nutrition Conference, Lillehammer, Norway (1996–99); and president of the Federation of European Nutrition Societies (FENS) (1999–2003). See Helsing and Häggkvist (2009); Helsing and Savage (1982). See also Figure 2.

Dr Edmund Hey

DM DPhil FRCP (b. 1934) trained as a respiratory physiologist in Oxford and worked for the MRC with Kenneth Cross, Geoffrey Dawes and Elsie Widdowson for some years before moving to Newcastle for a grounding in paediatrics in 1968. He established a respiratory intensive care service at Great Ormond Street Hospital, London, in 1973, before returning to Newcastle to set up a network of neonatal services for the north of England in 1977. Epidemiology, neonatal pharmacokinetics, and the conduct of controlled clinical trials have been his main research since his retirement in 1994.

Professor Peter Howie

MD FRCOG FRSE (b. 1939) trained in obstetrics and gynaecology at the University of Glasgow and was senior lecturer there (1974–78). At the MRC reproductive biology unit in Edinburgh as clinical consultant he developed a major interest in breastfeeding research (1978–81). He moved to chair of obstetrics and gynaecology at the University of Dundee (1981–2000) and became dean of faculty and deputy principal; held positions with WHO as task force chairman and was chair of the Scottish Council for Postgraduate Medical and Dental Education (1996–2002).

Professor Derrick (Dick) Jelliffe

(d. 1992) qualified in medicine at the Middlesex Hospital, London, and worked as an academic paediatrician in Sudan and Uganda as a district medical officer. He was professor of paediatrics at University College, Ibadan, Nigeria (1948–52); senior lecturer in paediatrics at the University College of the West Indies (1953/4), the University of Calcutta (1954–56) and in New Orleans, Louisiana (1956–59). He was UNICEF professor of paediatrics and child health at the University of East Africa, Kampala, Uganda (1959–66), before his appointment as director of the new Caribbean Food and Nutrition Institute, University of the West Indies, established by the Pan-American Health Organization. He moved to a chair in public health and paediatrics at the School of Medicine, University of California Los Angeles (1972–90) and directed the international health programme there (1989–91); and was founder editor of the *Journal of Tropical Paediatrics*. See Laurence (1994); additional information from Professor John Waterlow, 27 November 2000 and Professor Gerry Shaper, 6 December 2000. See also Trowell and Jelliffe (1958); Williams and Jelliffe (1972).

Professor Patrice Jelliffe

(d. 2007) a nurse and later laboratory technologist, was at the Makerere University in the 1960s with her husband Derrick Jelliffe. She took higher degrees in public health and was appointed to a chair at the University of California, Los Angeles. See Jelliffe and Jelliffe (1978); Latham (2007). See also www.waba.org.my/pdf/Tributo_a_ Pat_Jelliffe.pdf (visited 11 August 2008); Figure 2.

Professor Alan McNeilly
PhD DSc FRSE (b. 1947) trained in agricultural science at Nottingham and Reading with a doctorate in lactation at the National Institute for Research in Dairying, Shinfield with Professor John Folley and Dr Alfred Cowie. He joined the department of reproductive medicine, St Bartholomew's Hospital, London, in 1971 and developed radioimmunoassays for human prolactin and gonadotrophins for clinical application with Professors Tim Chard and Mike Besser. After a sabbatical in Winnipeg, Canada (1975/6), he joined Roger Short and David Baird in the MRC reproductive biology unit, Edinburgh, in 1976, to study lactational amenorrhea with Peter Howie. He has been a principal investigator in the renamed MRC human reproductive sciences unit in Edinburgh, since 1984. He was editor in chief, *Journal of Endocrinology* (1995–2000); chairman of the Society for Reproduction and Fertility (1994–2004); Dale medalist of the

Society for Endocrinology (2008) and Marshall medalist, Society for Reproduction and Fertility (2008).

Professor Kim Michaelsen
MD DrMedSci (b. 1948) has been professor of paediatric nutrition at the department of human nutrition, faculty of life sciences, University of Copenhagen; senior consultant at the paediatric nutrition unit at Rigshospitalet, University of Copenhagen, since 1998, heading a research group working with paediatric and international nutrition focusing on the short- and long-term effects of nutrition in early life in industrialized and developing countries. He was president of the International Society of Research in Human Milk and Nutrition (2004/5).

Mrs Rachel O'Leary
MA PGCE IBCLC (b. 1949) was accredited as a La Leche League (LLL) leader in 1980 and continues to support mothers learning to breastfeed in paid and voluntary posts. She has served in LLL publications departments and on the LLLI board of directors, as well as organizing local mother-to-mother support groups. She is employed by Cambridge University Hospital Trust and by children's centres in Cambridge and is a member of the board of directors of Baby Milk Action.

Professor Thomas Ernest Oppé
CBE FRCP (1925–2007) qualified at Guy's Hospital, did his National Service in the Royal Navy and trained at Great Ormond Street Children's Hospital, Harvard and St Mary's. He was a lecturer in child health, University of Bristol (1956–60); consultant paediatrician, United Bristol Hospitals, 1960; assistant director (1960–64) and director (1964–69) of the paediatric unit, St Mary's Hospital Medical School, consultant paediatrician, St Mary's Hospital (1960–90) and professor of paediatrics, University of London, at St Mary's Hospital Medical School (1969–90), later emeritus. He was consultant adviser in paediatrics, DHSS (1971–86), member, DHSS committees on safety of medicines (1974–79), medical aspects of food policy COMA (1966–88); chairman of the panel on child nutrition, COMA; child health services, (1973–76). See Oppé (1961).

Ms Gabrielle Palmer
MSc HumNut (b. 1947) set up the UK action group, Baby Milk Action, in 1980 and has worked with this organization for ten years. She published *The Politics of Breastfeeding* (1989), a key text for advocates for safer infant feeding practices. She joined Dr Felicity Savage as co-director of the breastfeeding: practice and policy course in 1992, Institute of Child Health, UCL. In 1999 she was appointed HIV and infant feeding officer for UNICEF. She was a lecturer in the public health nutrition unit at the London School of Hygiene and Tropical Medicine (2001–07), and serves on the UNICEF UK Baby Friendly designation committee (2007–09).

Dr Malcolm Peaker
DSc FRS FRSE (b. 1943) graduated in zoology from the University of Sheffield and was a postgraduate student at the University of Hong Kong. He joined the Institute of Animal Physiology, Babraham Institute, Babraham, Cambridge, in 1968; was appointed to the Hannah Research Institute, Ayr, in 1978, first as head of physiology and subsequently as director and Hannah professor in the University of Glasgow (1981–2003).

Dr Ann Prentice
OBE PhD (b. 1952) read chemistry at Oxford University, medical physics at Surrey University and natural sciences at Cambridge University. She has worked for the MRC since 1978, researching the nutritional requirements of women and children with projects based in Gambia, China and the UK. She has been director of the MRC collaborative centre for human

nutrition research in Cambridge since 1998. She sits on the UK scientific advisory committee in Nutrition and was president of the Nutrition Society (2004–07).

Professor Mary Renfrew

RGN SCM PhD (b. 1955) graduated from the University of Edinburgh in 1975, qualified in nursing in 1977 and in midwifery in 1978, and gained her PhD working on breastfeeding with the MRC reproductive biology unit, Edinburgh in 1982. She established the national midwifery research initiative at the national perinatal epidemiology unit in Oxford (1988–1994); was professor of midwifery at the University of Leeds (1994–2003), and has been professor of mother and infant health at the University of York since 2003. She established and directs the multidisciplinary mother and infant research unit (1996–); wrote a series of reviews of breastfeeding published by the Cochrane Library, the WHO Reproductive Health Library, the HTA programme, the DoH and NICE; and has been chair of the WHO maternal and newborn health strategic committee.

Mrs Patti Rundall

OBE (b. 1950) trained as an artist and teacher at Camberwell School of Art and Goldsmith's College, London, but switched careers, prompted by Gabrielle Palmer, to work on the baby food issue and she has been policy director of Baby Milk Action since 1980. She is a leader of the international Nestlé boycott, active in 20 countries; a coordinator of IBFAN's campaign to strengthen EU legislation on baby foods; a trustee of Sustain and on the secretariat of the Baby Feeding Law Group, a coalition of UK health professional and lay organizations.

Ms Ellena Salariya

RGN RM (b. 1931) trained in nursing and midwifery at Dundee and Glasgow; gained an MPhil at Abertay University and Ninewells Hospital and Medical School, Dundee. She has been a midwife in maternity wards, labour suites and the community in Dundee and latterly was post-graduation education and research officer at and Ninewells Hospital (1982–93). Her published work covers breastfeeding patterns; umbilical cord care; smoking habits in hospitalized antenatal women; development of a stool colour comparator; gut transit time of meconium in the breastfed infant in relation to weight loss; and the development and testing of a tool to measure the mother–child relationship during the first five days of life. See also Royal College of Midwives (1988).

Dr Felicity Savage

FRCP FRCPCH FFPH (b. 1939) worked in community child health in Zambia, Indonesia and Kenya (1966–84); as a medical officer with WHO specializing in policy development and training in breastfeeding (1993–2001); an honorary senior lecturer at the Institute of Child Health, UCL, and director of the breastfeeding practice and policy course; and has been chair of World Alliance for Breastfeeding Action since 2006.

Professor Roger Short

AM ScD FRCVS FRCOG FAA FRS (b. 1930), reproductive biologist, was lecturer, then reader at the University of Cambridge (1956–72); director of the MRC unit of reproductive biology, Edinburgh (1972–82); professor at the department of physiology, Monash University, Melbourne, Australia (1982–95); professorial fellow, department of obstetrics and gynaecology, University of Melbourne, Australia (1996–2005); and has been honorary professorial fellow, faculty of medicine, University of Melbourne, Australia, since 2006.

Dr Mary Smale

PhD (b. 1943) trained as a teacher and works as a voluntary breastfeeding counsellor for the National Childbirth Trust. She was an honorary research fellow in the mother and infant research unit, University of Leeds and has authored and co-authored several chapters and papers. She has published a pack to help with the training of breastfeeding supporters (Smale (2004)).

Dr Alison Spiro

PhD MSc RHV RGN (b. 1949) trained as a nurse in 1971 and a health visitor in 1973; worked as a voluntary breastfeeding counsellor for the National Childbirth Trust (1977–2007); has been a health visitor in Harrow since 1984 and has published in the nursing press. She completed an MSc in medical anthropology in 1994, studying breastfeeding in the Gujarati community, she continued these studies for a PhD in social anthropology and has carried out field work in Harrow and India. She is also a specialist health visitor lead for breastfeeding in Harrow and Northwick Park Hospital.

Dr Penny Stanway

(b. 1946) trained in general practice and worked in child health in Croydon (1971–76), becoming a senior medical officer. Since then she has written many books for the public on breastfeeding, childcare and nutrition and edited and contributed to various health partworks and encyclopaedias. She was health columnist for *Woman's Weekly* for 15 years and is on the professional advisory board of the La Leche League.

Jenny Warren

OBE RGN RM HV (b. 1946) worked as a nurse, midwife and health visitor before taking up post as coordinator to the Scottish Joint Breastfeeding Initiative (1992–95), then national breastfeeding adviser for Scotland (1995–2005); she worked as a voluntary counsellor and tutor for the National Childbirth Trust and later as breastfeeding supporter for the Breastfeeding Network. She also acted as consultant and course tutor to the UNICEF UK Baby Friendly Initiative as well as serving on its various committees. She was appointed OBE in 2000 for her work to encourage breastfeeding.

Professor Lawrence Weaver

MD DSc FRCP FRCPCH (b. 1948) was educated at Cambridge and St Thomas' before a career in paediatrics. He developed a special interest in infant nutrition at the MRC Dunn nutrition unit, Addenbrooke's Hospital, Cambridge, and Harvard Medical School (1984–93), before moving to the University of Glasgow as reader in human nutrition and has been the Samson Gemmell professor of child health there since 1996. He is also a senior research fellow in the

Wellcome Centre for the History of Medicine, University of Glasgow.

Mr John Wells

BSc Nutrition (b. 1944) graduated from the University of London in 1966 and started his career as a Voluntary Service Overseas officer in Guyana, where he participated in a WHO project. On returning to the UK he joined H J Heinz Co. where he initially worked as an analytical research chemist and was later appointed as company nutritionist. In 1980 he moved to Cow & Gate where he worked on the formulation and clinical assessment of baby milks intended for infants with special dietary requirements and also on updating the recipes of infant weaning foods. He served on a DoH committee advising government on aspects concerning the nutritional assessment of infant formulae (1995/6) and worked on scientific communication projects with staff at the Nutricia head office in both Friedrichsdorf and Amsterdam (1999–2006).

Professor Brian Wharton

DSc FRCP FRCPCH (b. 1937) graduated in medicine at Birmingham in 1960. While training as a paediatrician his first nutritional paper concerned the feeding of preterm babies. He spent two years at the MRC unit in Uganda studying kwashiorkor, the subject of his MD thesis. Subsequent paediatric posts were at the Institute of Child Health, University of Bristol; the Queen Elizabeth Hospital for Children, Great Ormond Street Hospital, Institute of Child Health, UCL (1969–73); the Sorrento Maternity Hospital Birmingham (1973–88); and King Fahd University, Riyadh, Saudi Arabia (1984). He was the foundation Rank professor of human nutrition at the University of Glasgow (1988–92) and director of the British Nutrition Foundation (1994–97). He is part-time honorary professor at the MRC childhood nutrition research centre, Institute of Child Health, UCL, and honorary research fellow at the Institute of Child Health, Birmingham.

Professor Roger Whitehead

CBE FBiol (b. 1933) joined the scientific staff of the MRC in 1959, becoming director of the MRC child nutrition unit in Kampala, Uganda, in 1968. He was director of the MRC Dunn nutrition centre at Cambridge and at Keneba, Gambia (1973–98). See Whitehead (1969).

Dr Anthony Williams

DPhil FRCP FRCPCH (b. 1951) trained in medicine at University College and Westminster Hospital Medical School, University of London, graduating in 1975. He was appointed research fellow in the department of paediatrics, University of Oxford, in 1980 following initial paediatric training in London, Leicester and Liverpool. In 1985 he moved to the University of Bristol as lecturer in paediatrics and has been a consultant paediatrician at St George's, University of London, since 1987.

Ms Carol Williams

is a public health nutritionist and infant feeding specialist. She trained originally in agricultural botany at the University of Reading, but moved into public health nutrition after working for the Voluntary Service Organization in Kenya. She has worked in emergency relief, health promotion and consumer advocacy and, since 1993, has combined consultancy work with part-time university teaching. She is co-director of the WHO/UNICEF collaborative breastfeeding practice and policy course at the Institute of Child Health, UCL, and teaches nutrition policy and infant feeding modules at the University of Westminster, London School of Hygiene and Tropical Medicine and Brighton and Sussex Medical School. She has worked as a trainer and consultant on infant feeding internationally, for UNICEF, World Alliance for Breastfeeding Action and Emergency Nutrition Network. She is a member of a mother-led breastfeeding drop-in charity, and the breastfeeding strategy group, Brighton and Hove.

Dr Cicely Williams

CMG FRCP (1893–1992), paediatrician and nutritionist, was the first paediatrician appointed to the Colonial Medical Service. See Dally (1968). The personal papers of Cicely Delphine Williams are held as PP/CDW in archives and manuscripts, Wellcome Library, London.

Dr Michael Woolridge

DPhil (b. 1950) trained in zoology and secured his DPhil in animal behaviour, supervised by Richard Dawkins. In 1979 he joined a multidisciplinary research team at the John Radcliffe Hospital, Oxford, co-directed by David Baum (paediatrics, Oxford) and Robert Drewett (psychology, Durham). In 1985 his research relocated to the Institute of Child Health, Bristol. He was the first national director of the UNICEF UK Baby Friendly Initiative (1993–95). Since 1996 he has been senior lecturer in infant feeding at the University of Leeds. All four of his children were successfully breastfed despite his intrusion.

Glossary[*]

Baby Milk Action

The UK member of the **International Baby Food Action Network,** responsible for co-ordinating the international Nestlé boycott.

Baby-friendly Hospital Initiative.

A worldwide programme of WHO and UNICEF, established in 1991, to encourage maternity wards and clinics to implement the *Ten Steps to Successful Breastfeeding* (www.unicef.org/newsline/tenstps.htm) and to practise in accordance with the *International Code of Marketing of Breast-milk Substitutes* (WHO (1981b)). The UNICEF UK Baby Friendly Initiative began in 1992 and was formally launched in 1994. Its principles were extended to community healthcare services in the *Seven Point Plan for the Promotion, Protection and Support of Breastfeeding in Community Health Care Settings* in 1998 (www.babyfriendly.org.uk/pdfs/Community_Initiative_Review_consultation_document.pdf). See www.babyfriendly.org.uk/page.asp?page=11 (all visited 17 June 2008).

Bellagio Consensus

The conclusion reached at a meeting of scientists in Bellagio, Italy, in 1988, sponsored by Family Health International, the Rockefeller Foundation, and WHO, that breastfeeding provides more than 98 per cent protection from pregnancy during the first six months postpartum if the mother is fully or nearly fully breastfeeding. The experts urged family planning providers to offer women the option of using breastfeeding to space births and to delay the use of other contraceptives (Family Health International (1988)). A second conference in Bellagio, 11–14 December 1995, sponsored by WHO, Family Health International, and the Georgetown University institute for reproductive health, and supported by the Rockefeller Foundation, reviewed research to test the 1988 consensus and concluded in its favour. See Kennedy *et al.* (1989); Short *et al.* (1991); Heinig (1998); www.who.int/reproductive-health/hrp/progress/55/news55_1.en.html; www.fhi.org/en/RH/Pubs/booksReports/LAMconsensus.htm (both visited 14 February 2009).

[*] Terms in bold appear in the Glossary as separate entries

The Breastfeeding Network

A UK-wide voluntary organization, established in 1997 to provide independent information and support to breastfeeding mothers and those involved in their care. It trains peer supporters, offering externally moderated training with the Open College Network. Together with the Association of Breastfeeding Mothers it operates the national breastfeeding helpline launched in February 2008, in addition to the Breastfeeding Network's own helpline which had 20 000 calls last year. Other services include a drugline, a drugs in breast-milk helpline and supporterline in Bengali/Sylheti. See www.breastfeedingnetwork.org.uk (visited 8 January 2008).

confounding variables

The association of a disease and a study factor with a third variable causing a spurious difference between cases and controls.

Convention on the Rights of the Child

The first legally binding international document to incorporate the full range of human rights – civil, cultural, economic, political and social – to children. It was adopted by the General Assembly of the United Nations by its resolution 44/25 of 20 November 1989 and came into force on 2 September 1990. It was ratified by the UK on 16 December 1991. Article 43 established a Committee on the Rights of the Child, which first met in October 1991 and currently holds three sessions a year, supported by the United Nations Centre for Human Rights in Geneva. See www.unhchr.ch/html/menu3/b/k2crc.htm; www.unicef.org/crc/; www2.ohchr.org/english/bodies/crc/index.htm (all visited 15 February 2009).

gonadotropin-releasing hormone

A 10-amino acid protein that is produced in the hypothalamus and acts on cells in the anterior pituitary to stimulate secretion of luteinizing hormone and follicle-stimulating hormone. It plays a pivotal role in the regulation of reproduction. See www.hrsu.mrc.ac.uk/glossary.php (visited 4 August 2008).

International Baby Food Action Network (IBFAN)

Formed in 1979 by six of the groups present at the WHO/UNICEF meeting on infant and young child feeding (1979), IBFAN is an umbrella organization with more than 200 citizen groups in more than 100 countries that monitor the baby food industry to strengthen controls on its marketing in accordance with the *International Code of Marketing of Breast-milk substitutes*.

La Leche League International (LLLI)

A private voluntary organization, established in 1956 by seven women who met to support each other in mothering through breastfeeding. Registered as a not-for-profit organization in Illinois, the network has now grown to include groups in over 60 countries. Accreditation is valid world-wide. Volunteer leaders offer breastfeeding counselling one-to-one by phone, in person and by e-mail, facilitate local mother-to-mother support groups, assist at drop-ins and breastfeeding cafés and can provide classes and sessions for antenatal education. Publications include *The Womanly Art of Breastfeeding*, journals for parents and health professionals, and information sheets on many topics. See www.lalecheleague.org (visited 8 January 2008).

La Leche League Great Britain

An affiliate of **LLLI**, with about 100 groups currently in GB, and over 200 leaders. Since the 1970s these groups have encouraged and supported many thousands of women to meet their own personal breastfeeding goals, overcome difficulties, enable babies to begin solid foods around the middle of the first year of life and to continue the breastfeeding relationship for as long as they wish to.

lactation

Requires two physiological mechanisms: milk secretion and milk ejection. Secretion is controlled by the release of prolactin from the anterior pituitary in response to the stimulus of suckling; the ejection is a neuroendocrine reflex when oxytocin is released from the posterior pituitary in response to suckling, which causes the contraction of the alveoli of the breast and release through the mammary ducts and nipple. See McNeilly and McNeilly (1978).

lactoferrin

An iron-binding protein found in human (and other mammalian) milks. It protects against infections by depriving bacteria of iron, which is an essential element for their proliferation and function.

MRC reproductive biology unit, Edinburgh (CRB)

Established in 1972 at the Queen's Medical Research Centre, Edinburgh, comprising the division of reproductive and developmental sciences (school of clinical sciences and community health, college of medicine and veterinary medicine) and the MRC human reproductive sciences unit. In 1989 it became a WHO collaborating centre and has strong links with the reproductive medicine laboratory in the adjacent

Royal Infirmary of Edinburgh.
See www.crb.ed.ac.uk/about.php
(visited 7 January 2008)

National Childbirth Trust (NCT)

An association of interested parents
and healthcare professionals,
started in 1956 when Prunella
Briance placed an advertisement
in the personal columns of *The
Times* and *The Daily Telegraph*
suggesting the formation of an
association to promote and better
understand the system of natural
childbirth described by Dr Grantly
Dick-Read (1890–1959) (Dick-
Read (1942)). The responses
became the nucleus of the Natural
Childbirth Association, later
becoming the National Childbirth
Trust, to which charitable status
was granted in 1961. See www.
nctpregnancyandbabycare.com/
about-us/who-we-are/history
(visited 6 August 2008).

National Dried Milk

The National Dried Milk scheme
was introduced in December
1941, a month after liquid milk
was rationed. It was available for
children under one year of age and
later to those under two years. It
continued to be sold in tins until
1976, being subsidized to those on
benefits in the 1960s and was used
for infant feeding.

Oppé Report, 1974

The DHSS Committee on Medical
Aspects of Food Policy (COMA)
Panel on Child Nutrition convened
a working party on infant feeding
in 1971, under the chairmanship
of Professor Tom Oppé. Other
members were: Professor G C
Arneil, Dr R D G Creery, Dr J
K Lloyd, Professor C E Stroud,
Dr Brian Wharton and Dr Elsie
Widdowson, with Dr D H Buss,
Miss D M Radford and Dr E M
Ring as assessors. It published its
first report in 1974, unanimously
recommending that the 'best food
for babies is human breast-milk',
and feeding in this way for four
to six months' duration would
'safeguard the infant from the
adverse conditions which are or
may be associated with artificial
feeding', but that even two
weeks' duration would offer a real
advantage. No universal cause for
the unpopularity of breastfeeding
was found, but cultural changes in
attitudes toward female sexuality,
motherhood and the role of
women were identified, along
with the provision and promotion
of artificial feeds. The report
recommended a survey of infant
feeding practices and stated that
working party members 'deprecate
the advertisement or promotion
of infant milks in any way which
suggests that a substitute milk is

equivalent or superior to breast-milk as a food for infants'. See DHSS (1974); Figure 3. A second report was published in 1980 (DHSS (1980)).

phenylketonuria (PKU)

A recessive disorder in humans associated with the inability to metabolize phenylalanine, usually due to the absence of phenylalanine hydroxylase, which causes raised levels of phenylalanine in the blood and impairs early neuronal development if not managed from the first weeks of life. The condition can be controlled by diet.

Rotersept (chlorhexidine)

A topical antimicrobial agent used in the treatment of mastitis, and as a general disinfectant in solutions, creams, gels and aerosols.

secretory IgA

An immunoglobulin (antibody) that protects mucosal surfaces, especially those of the gastrointestinal and respiratory tracts, against bacterial infections. It is secreted by the salivary glands and Brunner's glands, in the duodenum, and is abundant in human milk, especially in colostrum, which contains several g/L of IgA. Human milk IgA is important to the breastfed baby during the early months when its own ability to secrete this immunoglobulin is limited and developing.

Index: Subject

Index: Names

Biographical notes appear in bold

Key to cover photographs

Front cover, top to bottom
Professor Lawrence Weaver (chair)
Dr Elisabet Helsing
Dr Felicity Savage
Miss Chloe Fisher

Back cover, top to bottom
Professor Lars Hanson, Professor Brian Wharton
Ms Ellena M Salariya, Mrs Rachel O'Leary,
   Mr John Wells, Professor Roger Whitehead
Professor Anna Glasier, Professor Elizabeth Alder,
   Professor Roger Short
Professor Peter Howie, Professor Mary Renfrew,
   Professor Alan McNeilly

Printed in the United Kingdom by
Lightning Source UK Ltd., Milton Keynes
137399UK00001B/99-170/P